"Sally Maslansky's biograp. ⋯⋯ her therapeutic journey to comprehend and overcome the pervasive childhood trauma that led to her identity fragmentation, is truly inspirational. For survivors, Sally provides a sense of camaraderie, profound strategies, and insights, instilling hope for profound and embodied healing. Her description of her work with Dr. Dan Siegel serves as a masterclass for clinicians navigating and treating individuals with dissociative conditions, and may even offer vicarious healing to those experiencing such challenges."

—MARY-ANNE KATE, PHD, award-winning researcher in dissociation, trauma, and mental health; and member of the Scientific Committee of the International Society for the Study of Trauma and Dissociation (ISSTD)

"Sally Maslansky opens her heart and mind to share a deeply personal journey of self-discovery through the psychotherapeutic process. A heart-wrenching yet uplifting read, revealing how understanding and compassion shift suffering to authentic happiness."

—SUE SMALLEY, PHD, professor emerita in the department of psychiatry and biobehavioral sciences at the University of California, Los Angeles

"This book fills a much-needed gap in the self-help world! So many survivors of traumatic childhoods have dissociative identity disorder (DID) but suffer in silence needlessly. Thank you for helping to bring to light an often dismissed and stigmatized experience for so many! I will recommend this to clients and colleagues."

—KAYTEE GILLIS, LCSW, psychotherapist, and author of several books on childhood trauma, including *Breaking the Cycle* and *Healing from Parental Abandonment and Neglect*

"*A Brilliant Adaptation* is an extraordinary memoir. My wife Mary and I found it to be gripping from start to finish. A true page-turner that shook us to the core and drew deep, heart-rending emotions from both of us. Not your ordinary dry medical tome—far from it—and yet its story of surviving a childhood of severe physical and psychological trauma is a study of major importance. What incredible courage Sally Maslansky has in writing so truthfully as a person who lived through it, and as a skilled therapist who now treats others who have similarly suffered."

—FRED SCHEPISI, writer, producer, and director; and MARY SCHEPISI, artist and curator of auctions for The Australian Prostate Cancer Clinic

"Sally's story is one of extraordinary bravery, strength, and resilience in the face of unimaginable childhood trauma. Through it, we emerge with the valuable insight that we all have the capacity to work through our own trauma—Sally gives us the courage to do that. *A Brilliant Adaptation* is a page-turner. Despite being advised in the foreword to take it in slowly, I couldn't help myself—I at once read it through, cover to cover."

—KAREN BLUTH, PHD, associate professor emerita at the University of North Carolina, and author of *The Self-Compassion Workbook for Teens, The Self-Compassionate Teen,* and *Mindful Self-Compassion for Teens in Schools*

"Sally Maslansky's story of healing from early wounds is a testament to our capacity for transformation. This book reframes even the most fragmented inner worlds as places where hope, wholeness, and connection can take root and flourish. What an inspiration for all of us coming to terms with our lives as parents, as children, and as human beings."

—BETHANY SALTMAN, best-selling book coach, literary agent, and author of *Strange Situation*

a
brilliant
adaptation

HOW DISSOCIATIVE IDENTITY DISORDER & THE POWER OF THE THERAPEUTIC BOND SAVED ME

Sally Maslansky, LMFT

New Harbinger Publications, Inc.

Publisher's Note

This publication is designed to provide accurate and authoritative information in regard to the subject matter covered. It is sold with the understanding that the publisher is not engaged in rendering psychological, financial, legal, or other professional services. If expert assistance or counseling is needed, the services of a competent professional should be sought.

NEW HARBINGER PUBLICATIONS is a registered trademark of New Harbinger Publications, Inc.

New Harbinger Publications is an employee-owned company.

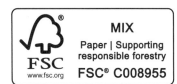

Copyright © 2025 by Sally Maslansky
New Harbinger Publications, Inc.
5720 Shattuck Avenue
Oakland, CA 94609
www.newharbinger.com

All Rights Reserved

Cover design by Sara Christian

Acquired by Elizabeth Hollis Hansen

Edited by Rebecca Job

The journal entry reproduced in part 3 of this book was also published in The Mindful Brain by Daniel Siegel, copyright © 2007 Daniel Siegel and W. W. Norton & Company.

Visit http://www.newharbinger.com/56944 to download a reading group guide for this book.

Library of Congress Cataloging-in-Publication Data on file

MIX
Paper | Supporting responsible forestry
FSC® C008955
www.fsc.org

Printed in the United States of America

27   26   25

10   9   8   7   6   5   4   3   2   1   First Printing

*For Sam, Paul, and Dan...for changing my life in all the ways
I always hoped that it would.*

Because this book contains explicit descriptions of childhood trauma and dissociation, I encourage readers to approach it with care. Taking breaks, reaching out for support, and initiating your own kinds of self-care are all useful as you engage with the material. Please keep in mind this is my personal story alone, not a reflection of anyone else's experience of trauma or DID. It's my offering of the possibilities of healing.

FOREWORD

WHAT A GIFT our courageous author has provided here in this life-affirming, deeply moving, and profoundly inspiring memoir about growing up in a troubled, terrifying home and building her way to a life of clarity, meaning, and connection. This unique offering reveals how our minds are shaped by our relationships, the traumatic ones early in life leading to a fracturing in how our emotions, thoughts, memories, and even sense of self can become disconnected as a "dissociative identity." This powerful adaptation of dividing the mind in order to conquer an overwhelming family experience also remains open to growth and change, through the healing power of relationships.

I have the deep privilege of both offering a few words reflecting on the importance of these insights into human development and being a therapist in connection with Sally Maslansky, our guide through this life-changing journey from fragmentation to wholeness. When we first met over a third of a century ago, Sally and I were of course younger, but the lessons her courage has taught me continue to inform and inspire my own professional work and personal life. Sally is a hero for me, showing us all how the capacity to grow toward mental health through the power of relational connections and inner reflection is a superpower each of us can harness across our lives.

First coming to me with her husband and newly adopted son, she later returned to see what "might be wrong" with her young child. The implicit sense that there was something "off" did not have explicit details in his child development—but it turned out to be a feeling inside that soon revealed a fragmented inner world that even Sally was not aware of inside herself. In this clear, concise, and compelling journey, we come to see how the impact of frightening experiences early in life at the hands of caregivers can lead to a fundamental way in which the usually connected processes of the mind, such as emotion, thinking, remembering, intention, and identity, can become disconnected from each other in a process known clinically as dissociation. In my own field of research training in attachment—how a child connects with caregivers—we had shown that one cause of dissociation is the experience in a family of the attachment figure being a source of terror.

Why would being terrified of your attachment figure—your mother, father, or other older (hopefully wiser), safe individuals—lead to such fragmentation of consciousness and the mind's overall functioning? One way to understand this empirically established finding is that the brain has two neural networks that become activated when a caregiver does something that intensely and repeatedly terrifies a child. One network is that of survival, which essentially says, "Get away from the source of terror"; in contrast, the other network says, "Go toward my attachment figure to be protected." Here, within one body, one drive is to go away and the other to go toward the same individual—the attachment figure who is the source of terror. This fear without solution leads to a disorganized attachment and a fragmentation of the mind's functioning. With early, repeated, and intense ruptures in the attachment relationship that go unrepaired, research reveals that one outcome is not only dissociation—feeling numb, not being able to recall certain experiences, disruptions in thought, feeling unreal—but also to a fragmented sense of identity.

Previously known as "multiple personality disorder" and then changed formally to "dissociative identity disorder," or DID, this condition is an adaptive response of the young child to terrifying, disorganized relational experiences. While the challenges to living a life of clarity and optimal regulation of emotions, thought, memory, and behavior are huge with those living with this situation as they grow into adolescence and adulthood, this is a disorder that is open to deep and lasting change.

When studies follow children exposed to early abuse or neglect known as developmental trauma, one of the main findings is that the ways in which differentiated areas are linked to one another—neural integration—is compromised. This is likely the source of the overall dysregulation with emotions and thought, and likely a component of the neural mechanisms underlying dissociation and dissociative identity disorder. Because of a lifelong process known as neuroplasticity, the brain remains open to growth in response to experiences so that it can change across the lifespan. As a therapist working within the framework of interpersonal neurobiology (IPNB), my aim is to harness the power of relational connections that are integrative—honoring differences while promoting compassionate linkages—in order to stimulate the neuroplastic growth of integration in the brain.

When we add the power of inner reflection to help guide neural firing toward integration alongside these sharings of energy and information flow (which are the essence of relational connections promoting integration and healing), we can see how the therapeutic bond combined with inner work can lead to profound transformation toward a more integrative, healthy mind. Sally's careful articulation of our relationship, our connection, and her inner work with various states of mind that had to be divided to help her survive a terrifying family reveals for us the important steps in this journey of transformation. Here you'll see how even if a family environment does not "make sense" in its chaotic and traumatizing way of negatively impacting development, an individual—with courage and therapeutic support—can come to make sense of the adaptations to a world that made no sense. Making sense is an integrative process, involving careful differentiation of emotion and memory, identity and meaning, and the sharing of that process in both consciousness within the individual and in communication in a close, therapeutic relationship.

I am deeply inspired by Sally's journey toward resolving her dissociative adaptation as well as her life-affirming capacity to articulate these steps for us all in this book. This is a story to take in slowly. Sit with its profound insights, explore its potential meaning for your own life and those you may know, and let this narrative of moving from fragmentation and survival to integration, coherence, and equanimity be an illuminating guide toward human flourishing. Thank you, Sally, for your courage to gift us your hard-earned life lessons. And thank you, dear reader, for taking the time to receive the gift of Sally's journey toward wholeness.

— Daniel J. Siegel, MD
Founder and director of education at the Mindsight Institute
Author of *The Developing Mind*, *Mindsight*, and *Mind*

DISSOCIATION: The process by which usually associated processes are dis-associated or compartmentalized from one another. Clinical dissociation can result in blocked access to memory and emotions, bodily numbness, or impairments to the continuity of consciousness across states of mind.

MAKING SENSE: A process of sorting through memory, here-and-now experience, and imagination such that we create a coherent picture of the essence of what is occurring in our lives. Making sense can be seen as an integrative process, linking past, present, and potential future in a way that enables these elements of thought, feeling, memory, and imagination to situate us in a social world of experience.

INTEGRATION: In general, the linkage of differentiated elements. The mind's process of linking differentiated parts (distinct modes of information processing) into a functional whole is postulated to be the fundamental mechanism of health. Without integration, chaos or rigidity ensues. Integration is both a process (a verb) and a structural dimension (a noun) and can be examined, for example, in the functional and anatomic studies of the nervous system.

All from *Pocket Guide to Interpersonal Neurobiology* by Daniel J. Siegel

PART 1

I COULDN'T EVEN REMEMBER how I got there. That was a little scary, because the route between my house in Malibu and his office in Brentwood was the Pacific Coast Highway—a notoriously tricky drive. Yet it was as if I'd driven there with my eyes closed.

What was I going to tell him? What would he ask me? So, so worried about Sam. *Is he okay? Will he be okay? Oh my god—what if he isn't going to be okay? Why am I so afraid? Why am I terrified all the time? What in fact is terrifying in my life? Being a new mother? Happily married? House on the beach? Beautiful life? What's wrong with me? What in the world's going on with me? Is he just going to tell me I'm crazy?* I felt a little crazy. And very nervous. Not so much about meeting him again, but about what he was going to tell me. I just had to figure these feelings out. *Please, please, please let Sam be okay.* And oh my god, the terror...and the tears...for god's sake, the tears.

"Hi, please come in."

"Thank you. Thank you, Dr. Siegel, for seeing me."

"It's nice to see you again—it's been just about a year, right?"

"Yes."

"How can I help you?"

Oh my—I do hope you can. Please, please, please be able to help me.

"Dr. Siegel, the thing is...I'm...oh boy. I'm really worried something is going on with Sam"—my son. "I mean, not now really—but, well, you see—well, there are these two books..."

1

I'd brought the two books with me: *On the Day You Were Born* and *The Family That Grew.*

"Do you mind if I read to you from these books? They were gifts to Sam. I think it's the best way to show you what's going on with me."

"Please do."

As I read them aloud to him, as if on cue, the tears began to pour from my eyes. Not just a trickle...a flood. It was crazy.

"And it happens every time I read them, Dr. Siegel."

"Every time?"

"Yes."

"Whenever I read them—to Sam, to Paul"—my husband—"to myself...just a flood of tears. Sometimes even just thinking about reading them. Tears, tears, tears."

"What does it feel like—reading them?"

Feel like? Like I'm crazy.

"I mean...I don't know. I mean, look at these books...they're all about being happy and how wonderful it is to be born and how much your family loves you and how beautiful the world is and isn't it great to be born and have a family...I mean, Dr. Siegel...how will I ever explain to Sam about where he came from? How can I explain that he was abandoned and spent the first sixteen months of his life in an orphanage in Romania? Won't hearing that do something terrible to him?"

Even though I'd put the books down, stopped reading them aloud, my tears were streaming...I just couldn't stop crying. And it was an odd kind of crying; tears, but no sounds...no gestures, no stuffy nose from crying—no noticeable signs of crying at all, except for the tears... oh, and wet Kleenexes I was clutching in my hands.

I was sitting in a chair just opposite Dr. Siegel. His face was full of compassion, and there was also a look of puzzlement—not skepticism, but deep curiosity. *What could this be about?* I imagined him thinking. *How can I help this poor woman?*

"You know, Sally, since you and Paul brought Sam to see me last year at the UCLA clinic, I've heard he continues to do well—that he's caught up developmentally to his age. I'm wondering if there's something going on with him that I'm not aware of?"

"I'm not sure what you mean?"

Again, compassion—but maybe a little confusion, too? I know I was confused.

"Well, I can see you're deeply concerned about Sam, but from all I know about his progress, it appears to me Sam's doing fine. I guess I'm just wondering what it is that's happening with Sam that has you so deeply concerned."

"I don't know exactly, Dr. Siegel. I mean, reading these two books all about love and family and gathering and happiness coming into the world...they just make me afraid and sad. How will I be able to explain to Sam how his life began? How can anyone ever understand life beginning like that? It makes me so sad for him. I love him so. I don't know how I'll ever be able to help him understand it. I'm hoping this is something you might be able to help me with." There was a question I just had to ask him. "Dr. Siegel—do you think I'm crazy?"

"No," he said. "No, Sally, I don't think you're crazy."

Driving home, I felt better. Not exactly sure why, but I knew he was going to help me understand what was going on. Help me be the best mom to Sam I could. I was excited about seeing him at our follow-up appointment next week. I'd hoped to see him sooner, but he was going to be away. He hadn't said he could help me, but the feeling I had was that he could and would. I was certainly ready. On the way home, I noticed that for the first time in a while, the fear and terror has subsided—a welcome reprieve. I felt I was about to begin a journey I'd welcome. It was the feeling of being in good hands.

No. No, Sally, I don't think you're crazy. His words were echoing in my mind. I would hold onto them until my next appointment.

I HATE THE INVISIBLE GAME.

Feels horrible. Scary, scary, scary. Tears, tears, tears...making everything worse. Silent tears. Mustn't-be-seen tears. Torture. I hate, hate, hate this game. I especially hate him. He's the meanest.

"Where'd Sally go?"

"She was just here a second ago."

"Where's...Ssssaaaalllllyyyyy...?"

"I am here! I am right in front of you!"

Was that my voice? Was I screaming inside or out? Both? Did anyone hear me?

"Wow—I wonder where she could have gone. Maybe I can have her dessert now if she is not here."

Please, please, please see me...

...alone in my bed, tears streaming, but terrified, knowing I would get in trouble for getting my pillow wet. So upset as I pass out in my clothes, meaning trouble for me in the middle of the night if the steps came to my door. Stinging across my whole body. I hate them. I hate them. I love them. I hate them. I need them. I love them. Ouch...ouch...ouch...please stop... please, please, please don't wet the bed...just a wet mess everywhere. Am I crying still? No one could hear me. I can't even hear me.

And then...poof...I disappear. Onto my tree. Not even cold out there. I'm gone. Tricky. Safe. Safe. Safe. Not me in there...no one even knows it's not me. It's her.

Invisible.

I HAD A NICE WEEKEND AT HOME with my husband, Paul, and with Sam, who was then two-and-a-half. Asking about my session with Dr. Siegel, Paul said it was a puzzle to him, too, that I was so concerned about Sam. Last year—September 1990—when we had brought Sam home from Romania at sixteen months old, he hadn't been walking or talking yet. Just two months later, when we met with Dr. Siegel at UCLA, Sam had started walking and developing sounds. Now, a year later at two-and-a-half, he was walking, talking, learning—a pure joy for us. Yet still, the fear and tears were never far from the surface for me, and I was looking forward to my next appointment with the doctor.

Back in his waiting room when he returned, I was so happy to be there, because I knew there was something missing that might explain my terror and I felt ready to explore it with him.

Sitting across from me again, he asked how I was feeling after our previous meeting.

"I feel good, Dr. Siegel. Paul and I talked, and he finds my concern for Sam puzzling too. Sam's made such progress. The joy he brings us as a toddler seems to contradict my fears. Paul reminded me to tell you about when the fear started."

"Oh good—would you like to tell me about that?"

I described the day we landed in Bucharest in June of 1990 on our way to the town of Sibiu, where we would meet Sam and begin the adoption proceedings.

"I don't remember being happier in my life! Here we were on the way to adopt our son. It was an amazing trip. Paul and I were filled with joy. Then as soon as I got off the plane, I was hit with this intense sense of danger. I noticed it right away but couldn't understand it."

"When you say you were hit with it—can you tell me more about how that felt?"

How it felt? I didn't so much feel it as *be* it. How did it feel? How did it *feel*? Why was that such a perplexing question for me?

"I just knew it. I felt kind of...frozen?"

I must've sat there for a few minutes—eyes closed, looking inside for the feelings. Who knew feelings would be so difficult to find, much less describe?

"It felt like something really bad was going to happen any minute."

"Could you feel it in your body?"

In my body? What does that mean?

"I don't think so."

"Was there any reason for you to be afraid?"

Well, we were in a country that six months earlier had had a bloody revolution. A country with a notoriously corrupt dictator and evil security force. Walking through customs, through the airport, checking into the hotel, and strolling through the city center, we noticed it was deafeningly quiet. People wouldn't look at you. It was strange. I was just scared.

"I didn't feel the fear—I *knew* the fear. Sounds weird to say—but it was a fear coming from inside me, not from outside. It wasn't so much a feeling—more like a premonition, or maybe even a state of mind—that something bad was going to happen. I don't know—it sort of felt like something always following me around."

"Did Paul feel it?"

"No. Not at all. And you know, I always feel safe with Paul. We spent much of 1989 in the Soviet Union where he was shooting a movie. Paul's a film producer and works all over the world—I never feel unsafe with him. But this time being with him didn't help. It felt like the one in danger was me—not him, not us. Just me. Kind of like... like I was in trouble..."

"With whom?"

"What?"

"Who did it feel you were in trouble with?"

His question threw me a little—I so often would feel I was in trouble, or about to be in trouble, and until this moment it hadn't occurred to me to wonder why I felt that. I think I just always believed I was in trouble. It could be for anything. I never knew what it would be. It felt like that most of the time. My whole life.

"I don't know. Just in trouble."

I asked him what he thought it all meant, and he answered in the way that now—especially as a therapist myself—always makes me smile inside. I wound up asking him the same question often, and I always knew his answer:

"Well, what do you think?"

I simply couldn't make sense of it. This very first time he asked me that, I went blank. Not in a scary way, but as if I was searching for an answer that wasn't there.

"I just don't know. Dr. Siegel. I'm feeling kind of blank, empty inside. I don't have a clue. You know, I often feel like I'm looking for answers that just aren't there."

He looked at me in a way I don't think anyone had ever looked at me before. His face was so friendly and kind, open to whatever was going on with me. No judgment. It felt like he was curious about whatever might be going on with me, even if it was nothing. I felt a tremendous sense of relief. I wasn't sure I'd ever felt that, or had any sense of what I was relieved *about*.

"I'm wondering, Sally, about your fears for Sam. And you've told me Paul is puzzled too, since Sam is fine. Sam is, in fact, flourishing. It has me thinking it might be worth exploring some things about your own childhood. I think it might help me to understand what's going on with you. How does that sound?"

"Oh, that sounds fine."

"Okay."

There was a pause. I wasn't sure what to say next. And nothing was coming to mind—again, that blank feeling.

"I'm not sure what you want me to talk about."

"Oh, well—can you tell me about your childhood, as far back in your childhood as you can remember?"

Another long pause.

He repeated his question.

"Can you tell me, Sally, what kind of childhood you had?"

I suddenly felt dizzy. Closing my eyes. Confused. Light-headed. I couldn't figure out why his question felt strange. Suddenly I had an awareness that something was changing. There was even a momentary feeling of terror. Why, why the terror?

"Um...well yeah..." opening my eyes..."I had a good childhood."

"Oh good."

"Yes."

"Can you tell me about it?"

The sensations—even stranger now.

"I'm not sure what you mean."

Here he paused. The same look of understanding, but mixed with some—not really confusion—curiosity?

"Well, you've told me you had a good childhood."

"Yes."

"Can you tell me something good about it?"

I wasn't sure how to answer, because I didn't quite understand his question. I was having trouble taking it in. Like something lost in translation. I was feeling a little...kind of...how do I say it...out of body. I think he might've noticed.

"You know, Dr. Siegel...the thing is...I don't...um...well, I don't really remember my childhood."

He shifted in his chair and looked at me with the kindest expression and said, very gently...

"How do you know it was good then?"

For a moment, it felt like I left not just my body, but the room. It felt like a brief departure, but it must've been for longer than I thought because our one-hour session was almost over, and it seemed to have zipped by.

"What are you thinking?" he asked me...and his look was—I can't really describe it, except it made me feel safe and connected to him.

"I don't know, Dr. Siegel. I mean, I don't know what's worse—that I'm thirty-seven and don't remember my childhood, or that I'm thirty-seven and just realizing that it might be important."

We sat there for a moment or two. Our time was up, but I think he wanted to make sure I was okay to drive. I must've looked as disoriented as I felt. He had me take some breaths to ground myself, and before I left, I asked, "Is it possible to see you tomorrow?"

"Yes—yes, I could see you at nine o'clock. Will that work?"

I left his office feeling okay, knowing I'd be back in less than twenty-four hours.

I LET PAUL KNOW A LITTLE BIT about my session with Dr. Siegel. It was the first time he told me he'd always thought it strange I didn't remember much about childhood. Whereas I thought it was remarkable he remembered so much about his. Growing up in New York City—playing in the street and being run over—twice—by a taxi! Growing up with two brothers he loved. His dad being in the war, his mother's affair, his parents' divorce, how afraid he was of his mother and how much he loved and admired his dad. Not all his memories reflected a perfect childhood, but I loved hearing them. He was close to his brothers, too—they often spoke daily. Connected. I marveled at how many memories they shared, and how much they loved to talk about them, over and over again. And he was close to friends he'd known since he was born—they were his closest friends, and they had a lot of shared memories, too. We saw them often. Traveled together. Knew each other's families and friends. It was a whole new world to me. I loved spending time with them, hearing their stories. There was a familiarity among them that felt so warm and inviting. They were connected to each other in ways I'd never experienced.

But as much as I admired it, enjoyed being part of their story now, I'd never thought about it—friends, family, deep connectedness—as something missing for me. I somehow never wondered why Paul remembered so much and had such close relations with friends and family, while I had no memory of childhood, and no close connections to family or friends from before high school.

Looking back now, I believe that sense of connectedness is one of the things I loved most about Paul from our first meeting. Even if it hadn't occurred to me that I didn't have any of those connections or memories, I must've sensed that he possessed something I was missing.

BACK IN DR. SIEGEL'S OFFICE early the next morning, I opted for the couch instead of the chair opposite him.

"I'm wondering how you're feeling about our session yesterday," he began.

"I don't know, Dr. Siegel. I just don't know, or understand...it seems so odd, not that I don't remember my childhood, but that it's never seemed important to me before."

I told him about my talk with Paul and how he'd said that he'd always thought it strange that I remembered so little.

"What do you think it means?" I asked.

And of course, his reply,

"We don't know what it means yet. Can you tell me what it means to you?"

"I think that it's what I'm here to figure out. I've been really thinking about our session yesterday—about what it's like to feel so disconnected. I say I feel it, whatever 'it' is—but I'm not sure what that means."

"Not sure what it means?"

This really took me aback. It wasn't unlike what happened when we landed in Romania. Not so much a feeling, but maybe a total lack of feeling, in the midst of some awareness that something bad was going to happen. Like a warning...*Better go blank so you won't remember anything.*

"I'm not sure what it means to feel. It's not so much that I feel empty—but that I *am* empty. I don't know if I have any memories."

I didn't have one inkling of a memory about my childhood. Well, I could picture the houses I lived in—even their floorplans. I could remember my dogs. I knew I had siblings, five, and I knew who they were and how I felt about them. I don't remember much about the sister who was two years older than me, or the brother ten years older—just that I didn't like being around them much. My oldest sister, twelve years older, I loved, could count on. The only brother I liked, fifteen years older, I liked being around, though he was hard to know. And the oldest brother, seventeen years older, I never really knew. I thought he was kind of cool when I was a teenager because he smoked and did drugs, but he made me uncomfortable in other ways. But it wasn't like I knew anything about any of them—I just knew how I felt in their presence. Uncomfortable. I couldn't conjure up even one memory about any of them. No sense of connection, only a strong drive to stay clear of the two closest to me in age. Except for going to see *Sleeping Beauty* with my oldest sister when I was five, I didn't remember one fun time with any of them—couldn't recall anyone laughing, or doing or saying anything connecting me to them. Unlike how Paul was connected to his siblings, I couldn't tell one story about growing up with any of them.

I had no memories of feeling connected to anyone much earlier than high school. I could remember some friends from elementary school and junior high, when we lived in Chapel Hill, and had some good memories of them, but I hadn't seen or communicated with them since the end of ninth grade when we moved to Galveston.

"I'm disconnected from me. From life before I met Paul about ten years ago. I know about my life now—I know the people in my life, who they are, and I do love them and feel connected. But when you ask me what I'm feeling—I don't know that I feel anything. I can think about people, but I don't feel much. Except numb. I feel numb. Head to toe."

"How about to Paul?"

"I feel connected to Paul."

"Can you elaborate on what that feels like? What it feels like to be connected to Paul?"

"It feels like I know him, and he knows me. I'm never afraid of Paul. Ever. I feel safe with him. We have a great life. Our life together, especially now with Sam, gives me so much meaning. We have so much fun. Even when we disagree or fight, we manage to work things through. I'm happy to be married to Paul. I love him."

"How about to Sam?"

"Oh yes. I love Sam deeply. I want to spend every moment with him. I want to take care of him. I want him to have a wonderful childhood. I guess I mean…What do I mean? I feel connected to Sam and Paul. But I'm not sure I feel connected to myself. I can't describe that feeling—but it is odd. It unsettles me now, as I'm thinking about it."

Dr. Siegel was happy to know I felt connected to Sam and to Paul, and we ended the session soon after. Before I left, we made more appointments, agreeing for the next month or so to meet a few times a week with longer sessions. We settled on meeting three times a week, two hours each session.

AT THE BEGINNING OF OUR NEXT SESSION, Dr. Siegel asked, "What do you think, Sally, is the most robust predictor of how a child will do in life?"

I couldn't even imagine an answer.

"I've no idea."

"Research from the field of attachment tells us the most robust predictor of how children will grow up to thrive, not just survive, is the degree to which that child's parents have made sense of their own life story."

"Oh no—what does that mean for Sam? I mean...I know nothing about my childhood."

He paused, seeing how worried this made me.

"That's where we want to start, when you're ready. To dig deep, making sense of your story."

"How do we do that? How can I make sense of what I don't remember?"

I was feeling a little dizzy.

"Making sense is an integrative process, Sally—linking your past, present, and possible future by sorting through your memory, here-and-now-experience, and imagination. Working on having a coherent narrative of your life."

A coherent narrative of my life. *My story.*

"Making sense of my story—doing that will help Sam grow up to thrive, not just survive?"

"Yes, it will help Sam. It will help you help Sam. And it will help you."

"What if it's too late for me, Dr. Siegel?"

"It's never too late to make sense of your story, Sally—and there's no time like the present. That's what we're here to do together."

"What if it's too horrible to know?"

"Making sense, Sally, being able to know and tell your story, is what will free you from the constraints of your past—no matter what happened."

With that, we commenced with some questions that were the starting place of the journey of my lifetime—digging into the past, making sense of what happened, understanding how it impacted me today, knowing the truth of my story.

"The truth will set you free," he told me that day.

And it would—eventually.

"Let me ask you something, Sally...if you can, tell me some adjectives that describe your relationship with your mother as early as you can remember."

I heard that, but absolutely nothing came to mind. I sat there for a minute or two with my eyes closed. As I opened them, I had to ask him to repeat his question.

"Can you tell me some adjectives that describe your relationship with your mother—going back as young as you can?"

Blank. Empty.

"I can't think of one word. Nothing."

We just sat for a moment silently—then,

"How about for your father?"

"Terror."

Terror! The word leapt from my mouth before I'd even fully registered. I was stunned. I didn't feel out of body as the day before—I felt strangely present.

"Tell me what you're thinking, Sally?"

"I don't know."

He then asked me another question.

"Sally, when you were little and you were upset, who'd you go to for help?"

That question filled me with fear.

"I don't know. Nobody. Why am I feeling so empty yet so full of terror, Dr. Siegel? How can I not have any memories or feelings about my childhood? What's wrong with me?"

I just felt fucking crazy. *I think you're wrong, Dr. Siegel—I think I must be crazy.* I felt fucking crazy.

"What's going on?"

I don't fucking know.

I took a breath to steady myself. "I've got a lot of work to do. I want to figure this out."

And I knew who I wanted to talk to.

BACK IN DR. SIEGEL'S OFFICE after the weekend I was anxious to tell him about the conversation I'd had with my oldest sister. I'd told her about the work I was doing. That it turned out I had no memory of childhood. I'd asked if she thought something bad could've happened to me—did she know of anything bad that had happened to me? I mean, she was twelve when I was born and might have memories about me I didn't.

"She said the weirdest thing."

"Can you tell me?"

"She thought it was possible. No actual accounts. But it didn't seem out of the question. I mean, I was thinking, *she knows something I don't*. But then she said something, Dr. Siegel, that kind of freaks me out. It's weird."

"Can you tell me what she said?"

"She said, 'Well, I sure hope when you find out what happened, that it wasn't mom."

He looked a little startled.

"What do you make of that, Sally?"

I really didn't know what to make of it. It felt like some internal shift. What she'd said about our mom seemed out of left field. It made no sense to me. It made me dizzy.

"You know, Dr. Siegel, it feels like brain scramble."

"Tell me more about that if you can."

"Realizing at this stage of life I don't know anything about growing up is a shock. The one person I knew I could count on was my oldest sister. Talking to her about this was strange. I'm just...I mean..." I had to pause. "Oh boy. I hate this feeling."

"What feeling?"

"That I don't know who I am."

Or where the fuck I come from.

"Sometimes," I said, "leaving your office, I don't remember what we talked about. I know we talked—but it's fuzzy."

"Can you say more about that?"

"Not really. I just feel out of it a lot these days."

"Just since we've been meeting?"

I almost said yes, but I knew the feeling wasn't new.

"Not really. I mean, I think it happens sometimes. I feel...I don't know...not quite sure how to explain what I want to say...I'm not always aware of what's happened...sometimes even when something's going on, I'm not sure I'm there. It's...I don't know."

"I'd love to know more about that."

"It's like...kind of like I'm not always aware of what's happened, or happening...or that I've been here, or other places. I *know* something happened, or that I've been somewhere or done something, but the details sometimes...I mean, as you and I've been talking about childhood and how clearly I don't remember it, I realize I don't remember other things too. I know something occurred, I just have this...this vague awareness of it—not just about childhood, but about things I might've just done. It's weird."

"You know, Sally, my therapist, when I say something is weird, asks me to be clearer. Can you tell me more about this vague feeling that it's not just about childhood?"

"I know I had a childhood. And I know I do things. I know I see friends. But since I've been seeing you and realize I don't remember things from my past, sometimes I don't remember about now. And I want to ask you why you think that is, but I know you'll ask me what I think...and I just don't know."

"I don't know either, Sally. But I believe we'll figure it out together."

I went from sitting to lying on the couch, putting a pillow over my head. I wanted to scream. I'm sure Dr. Siegel could feel my frustration.

"I wish I could scream."

"It's okay—you can scream."

"I can't."

"It's okay."

"I don't know why. I've just got to keep it all in."

"You can scream into the pillow."

I wanted to scream, but the reality of doing it was something I couldn't imagine. Lying there with the pillow over my face—head spinning, world spinning—I felt frozen again.

"Someone might hear me."

"The only one who'll hear you is me, and I'm fine with you screaming."

Deep dive inside. Eyes closing. Head spinning with so many feelings. Oh god...the feelings. Physical feelings. Sad. Mad. Mostly the terror. Internal forces unleashed, vying for control. *No one can hear. Please, please, please don't let this happen. I can't do this here. Pray, pray praying: not here. The brave part. Crazy part. Afraid part. The part that knows. Parts that don't know. The-what-is-happening part. The this-can't-be-happening part. The don't-let-them-know part. Please, please, please don't let them know. The this-is-fucking-happening part. Internal tornado drilling a giant divide right down my middle. Tsunami pulling me down to the bottom. Heart pounding on one side. Stopped on the other. Words, thoughts, explanations, emotions, smells, and oh god...not the feelings...please, please, please STOP the feelings...I can't stand feeling that...I hate, hate, hate the feeling...I hate, hate, hate them. Oh no, oh no, oh no. He must be seeing this. Oh no, no no...not the terror. Please not the terror. Okay, okay, okay.*

Eyes pop open in terror.

We sat there for a moment or two. I knew where I was but couldn't figure out where I'd been or what just happened. Nothing was making sense. Fuck.

"What's going on, Sally?"

Silence, getting grounded. Takes time. Kind understanding face. Tears streaming.

"I just don't know."

Putting the pillow down.

"Did I scream?"

"No."

"Dr. Siegel, I don't know. Something's happening. I feel crazy. Terrified."

"You're not crazy."

"How can you tell?"

"I just know that's not what's going on here."

"Okay. But I'm terrified and I don't know why. It's inside of me and I need to know what it is."

OVER THE NEXT MANY WEEKS, we met regularly. Dr. Siegel took more history, though I continued to have no memory of childhood, just a sensation of terror. Feeling blank. I was still forgetting.

"Dr. Siegel, how can I not remember things but feel so much fear?"

He told me something so essential about how memory works.

"The brain encodes memory two ways—explicitly and implicitly. When your brain retrieves an explicit memory, it comes with a tag that lets you know it is from the past—it is not happening now. With implicit memory however, there is no tag—it is a visceral or behavioral response, and you think it is about what is happening now, not about something from your past."

"Like a memory of a feeling?"

"Exactly."

"So, the fear and terror might be memories of feelings from when I was little? A memory of feeling crazy and terrified as a kid?"

"They might be. We just don't know yet."

I had to really soak this in. Learning about implicit memory was the first time I began to understand the meaning of making sense. It wasn't just understanding what'd happened in my childhood, but understanding how things I'd experienced in childhood might continue to affect me in my present.

"Can you tell me what you're thinking, Sally?"

"Is implicit memory like a flashback—you know, like war vets experience?"

"Yes, implicit memory is most likely a building block of flashbacks."

Still taking this in. It made so much sense.

"Can you tell me what you're thinking?"

"About the times I might've been experiencing implicit memories."

"Can you tell me?"

I told him about how when I'd visit my parents' house after I was out of college—not a house I'd lived in—at night I would become overwhelmed with fear.

"I mean, so terrified I couldn't sleep. Really not sleep—not a moment's sleep."

"Do you know what you were afraid of?"

"Of being killed. Not being safe in bed. I couldn't figure out any reasons—there were no reports of escaped convicts or anything like that on the news. I'd just lie there, eyes wide open, waiting, paralyzed in fear...in bed...waiting for someone to come kill me."

Feeling it my body now.

"What's going on in your body?"

Frozen.

"I can't feel my body. Dr. Siegel, it feels like my body's not me."

"Can you tell me a little more?"

I didn't think I could. "Could we talk about something else?" I said. "I'm feeling dizzy."

My head was spinning.

"Of course we can. How dizzy—do you need to lie down?"

I was sitting on the couch and had my head hanging down.

"Why don't you lie down if you're feeling dizzy."

I did lay down and took some breaths. I wasn't just dizzy...it felt like I was balancing between two worlds and didn't know which way to lean. Scared, but also a little disconnected from the immediate feeling of fear. It was strange.

Dr. Siegel told me about something called a "dorsal dive." When your nervous system gets overwhelmed and starts to shut down, he explained, there can be a series of reactions—fight, flight, freeze, and feigning death—which can lead to fainting as a protective measure. That sounded exactly like what I was experiencing.

"How about if we use the rest of our time today, Sally, to get more family history?" he suggested. "Does that feel safe?"

"Yes—that sounds fine."

I felt in such good hands with him, but I wasn't quite ready to dig deeper. Getting some family history felt okay because I did remember certain things I'd been told about my family, and those were questions I thought I could answer.

"Do you know of any family history of mental illness?"

"How would I know if there was?"

"Was there ever any talk about people being crazy, or hospitalized? Any suicides?"

"How would I know if there were any suicides?"

"Did anyone in your family die under strange circumstances?"

I took my time and then remembered something: "There was a cousin."

I'd never known him; he was the son of one of my mother's siblings. I was the youngest in my family, and my mother was the youngest in hers, both by a lot of years. So, my cousins on her side were all fifteen or more years older than me. This cousin had died before I'd been born.

"He died?"

"Yes."

"How?"

"He accidentally hung himself in the closet when he was fourteen. And when I was a teenager I was always afraid that might happen to me."

As I said it, a wave of realization washed over me.

You don't fucking hang yourself by accident. In a closet. With a belt. I'm not even sure how I first heard that story. It was told so casually—I always took it as a cautionary tale, *don't go near any closets*— but it was told in passing, like anyone could accidentally hang themselves...in a closet. Like that could be an accident!

Over the next couple of weeks or so, I filled Dr. Siegel in on other family details. My mother had a sister who'd been committed. I didn't know any more than that. She'd been alive, I think, when I was a kid, but I'd never met her. The whole family seemed afraid of knowing about her. Or certainly afraid to talk about her. My dad's father I only remember meeting once—he died when I was just a little kid—and I didn't like him. I learned, I think in college (long after he died), that he'd been given a lobotomy. I think the story was that he'd burned the family house down, so he was given a lobotomy. And my oldest brother—he hadn't gotten a lobotomy, but the story goes that he was looking for a bug behind a curtain when he was a kid, lit a match so he could see better, and burnt the house down too. Another uncle—also someone I never met—died tragically, when his car got stuck on some railroad tracks, by accident, and he'd been hit by a train! (Again, reciting this, I thought, *Accident?*) And there was another cousin—I'd known him when he was an adult and I was in high school—who took a swim in the ocean and was never seen again.

As I told Dr. Siegel these stories about my family, what troubled me most was how it never occurred to me, until now, how strange they were, or how little they seemed to matter to anyone in my family. They never talked about these things as if they were terrible, or upsetting, or fucking crazy! No, they were just everyday events, barely worth mentioning outside the odd times they happened to come up. "As if they were no big deal, Dr. Siegel."

All of it was information, but none of it made sense. Real things happened to people. Real people suffered. Dr. Siegel and I had talked so much about the importance of making sense of our stories, but it seemed no one in my family was interested in doing that. The only sibling I felt comfortable reaching out to about any of this was my oldest sister, but she hadn't wanted to talk much since the hoping-it's-not-Mom conversation. It never occurred to me to reach out to the others. It was up to me. It had to be me going deep inside—into memory, disorientation, crazy stories and accidental hangings, feelings and memories of feelings—to find the answers. My answers. *I* had to make sense of it all.

A little time passed, and then Dr. Siegel suggested that, when I was ready, we could start with some deep relaxation and internal focus practices.

"Will it help me figure things out?"

"I think so."

I wasn't quite ready to take that next step...I knew eventually I would be. Just not quite yet.

Dr. Siegel was reassuring. "We can go as slow as you need to."

Going slow sounded good. As we continued to meet, we talked more about day-to-day life. Life at home with Sam and Paul was good. With them I felt the most grounded—stable and safe. Paul and I weren't talking a lot about my therapy sessions at home, but I'd let him know that they were about my not having the memories of childhood that he did; that that's what Dr. Siegel and I had been working on. And Paul had of course met Dr. Siegel when we'd taken Sam to see him at UCLA, and he liked him. He thought these sessions with Dr. Siegel were a good idea—he'd been so helpful in our understanding about Sam's development and the impact of his early childhood in the orphanage. Paul also knew I was struggling with some things and wanted me to find answers.

TAKE THE DAY, a few weeks later, that I showed up for our session, and when Dr. Siegel greeted me, he seemed—I couldn't quite tell if he was worried or confused. I went into his office, sat down, and started to talk, and he asked, "What time did you think we're meeting today?"

"Now—one o'clock."

He paused, and then said,

"No, Sally—we were scheduled for two hours at twelve."

"Really? Did we change it?"

"Yes—we spoke yesterday and changed it."

"I don't remember."

This felt awful to me. I'd never missed, cancelled, or confused any of our sessions. And I had no recollection of talking to him about rescheduling. I realized there'd been a few things like this lately—me feeling confused, disoriented, and even at times...lost. Late. Forgetful. My head was spinning, but not in the dizzy way. Tears flowed.

"Can you tell me what's going on now?"

I could hear the concern in his voice. Or not so much concern as... compassion. Caring. Connection.

"Dr. Siegel, I'm so confused. I just don't remember us talking."

"It's okay, Sally."

"I know—but it's not just that."

"What is it?"

"I just don't remember a lot lately."

"Tell me about that."

I'd been forgetting things the last couple of weeks—some friends mentioned I seemed to be a little out to lunch. I hadn't told anyone except Paul so far about what was going on in therapy.

"There's something I want to tell you Dr. Siegel, but I'm afraid to."

"Afraid of what?"

That you're wrong, Dr. Siegel. That I'm crazy. Or losing my mind. I'm upside down. I barely know where I am lately.

"That I'm having memory lapses."

He looked at me with an expression that was conveying something I can't quite describe. It brought up a feeling of connection and care so deep it nearly melted me, because I had never experienced anything like it. I knew he was there to help me. I knew he could help me. I knew he was helping me.

"I know you are, Sally."

"What do you mean? How do you know?"

He placed his notebook and pen on the footstool in front of his chair and leaned slightly toward me. He let me know that the last couple of sessions I'd come in not remembering what we'd spoken of last time. That I did at times seem disoriented and confused. He said once he wasn't sure I knew who he was or why I was there. He was so kind in his approach, and clearly not just concerned but invested in what was going on with me and as curious as I was. I felt that he would stick with me until we figured it out together. It was an extraordinary feeling for me. This was a sense of support I'd never experienced before. And while he showed his concern, he was completely matter-of-fact about it. I was able to remain grounded because he was so grounded.

Wow—he knew.

"Sally, we have some work to do...but we're going to have to wrap up. We'll pick this up tomorrow, and I'll share with you more of what I'm thinking may be going on."

"Dr. Siegel?"

"Yes?"

"I'm sorry I was late."

"I understand."

"Am I having a nervous breakdown?"

"I don't think that's what's going on with you, Sally."

"Can you tell me what you think is going on with me?"

"Not a nervous breakdown, Sally. I think you may, however, be on the verge of a nervous breakthrough."

"Breakthrough" sounded good. I was a little scared...but excited too. I knew he was right. I knew I was going to figure this out.

NEXT SESSION. "How are you feeling today?"

"You mean because of yesterday?"

"Yes."

"A little wobbly. But I'm glad I told you about it, and that you told me about me coming in and not really knowing why I was here. Before we dig into that, though, I need to tell you something."

"What's going on?"

"I've been having awful dreams. Upsetting nightmares. I can't sleep after. I'm afraid to go to sleep because of them."

"Tell me about that."

"I always feel like something really bad is going to happen."

"Do you want to tell me one of your dreams?"

"It's dark out...I'm riding my bike in Galveston, where I lived in high school. It was fun...my friends were behind me because I was going so fast...when I turned to look back...they were gone and suddenly...I was running fast, out of breath—a monster was chasing me! Not a monster like in a movie—a real-life monster, it was going to catch me. I was terrified, I thought I was about to die, I didn't want to see who it was, because I think I *knew* who it was and was afraid to know...like if they knew I knew...something bad would happen, and finally when I couldn't run anymore I stopped to look...and their face was blank and I woke up."

It felt scary telling it.

"That's some dream."

"What do you think it means, Dr. Siegel?"

"How about you tell me what it means to you?"

"What do you think dreams mean? Why do we have dreams?"

"One way to think about dreams, Sally, is they are a way the left and right hemispheres of your brain integrate things you are trying to make sense of."

"So, my brain is working on making sense of why I'm so afraid?"

"Yes, I think so. We've been working on your history and what it means—dreams may be one way your mind is working to make sense of it. Integrating it."

"How can I make sense of it if the dream won't let me see who I'm afraid of? It just lets me know I'm afraid, I already know that. I want to know what I'm afraid of. Who am I afraid of? How can I have no idea what or who is so terrifying?"

He asked if I was ready to try an internal focus practice to help me gain some insight into these difficult feelings. He explained he'd count down from ten to one, helping me relax and be grounded as I focused my attention on my internal world.

Relaxed.

Deeply grounded.

Focus of attention.

Internal world.

"How do you feel about trying it?"

"Okay." I took a breath. "What do I do?"

"Start by getting comfortable there."

I was sitting on the couch. He was in his chair facing me.

"Is it okay for me to lie down?"

"Sure—get comfortable."

I'd brought a blanket for his office to use when I was there—now three, sometimes four times a week. I put a pillow under my head, arranged the blanket over me, and held onto another pillow, which always made me feel a little better when I needed it.

"Okay."

"Ready?"

"Ready."

"Gently closing your eyes...I'm going to count down slowly from ten to one."

"What should I do?"

"Relax, listen to the sound of my voice, breathe."

Breathing in. Breathing out.

"Starting now at ten..."

I could already feel myself relaxing into myself in a way I hadn't experienced before. Eyes closed, but not dark—there was light coming through, as though someone had lit up the inside of my head. I couldn't quite make out the source of the light—it was just inside my head.

Breath slowing.

Relaxing.

"Down to nine..."

Noticing my body. Comfy on the couch. Cozy with the blanket. Hugging the pillow.

"Deeper down to eight..."

Relaxed and focused going deeper and deeper within. *Feels safe here.*

"To seven...six..."

Deeply relaxed. Such a good place to be, deep within myself. Knowing I'm here...going inside...Comfortable. Open. Curious. Safe.

Grounded.

"Five...four...three..."

Floating a little...still grounded...I like being here. Dr. Siegel's voice softer, and a little distant...

"Down even deeper at two..."

This is good.

"And stopping now at one..."

I'm here.

Focused.

Quiet for a little bit.

Breathing...

"Imagine, if you can, a hallway with doors."

"Okay."

I'm at the top of a hallway.

"Can you see the doors?"

The hallway is lined with doors.

"Can you find a door to stand in front of?"

I'm slowly going down the hallway, and I stop at a door. I'm just looking at it.

"It's feeling a little scary."

"Where do you feel the scary?"

My chest is tight—kind of like when you just start to think you might be getting a cold.

"It's a little hard to breathe—I'm not sure...not sure I can do this... it's feeling so hot."

"Taking your time..."

Taking in some steadying breaths...

"Okay—I'm in front of a door. What should I do now?"

"Can you open it?"

"No. I can't."

"Tell me more."

The terror welled up and I could barely speak. I must've been silent for a while. We were both silent.

"What's going on now?"

"I can't open the door, because the doorknob is turning red from the heat. The room is on fire. My skin feels on fire. It's too hot...It's too hot..."

It's so fucking hot.

"Please," I gasped. "Get me out of here."

It felt paralyzing. The terror was in full force and taking over. I could barely breathe. I wanted to flee. *No, Sally—stay...stay.*

"I hear it feels like it's on fire. But remember, it's a memory of a feeling. I'm here with you. We're safe. We're in my office—and I promise you nothing will burn."

I opened the door. Stumbling...tumbling. Once, when I was little, I almost drowned in the ocean. I hadn't really been afraid; I would've been okay with it. It wasn't until a wave pulled me under and turned me all around, and I couldn't tell top from bottom, that there was fear. Now, I was feeling that again—dizzy, tossing around—

And then I was breathing, and moving through the water...like a dolphin...I could see things...without being there...Poof. I was blank. Invisible. Gone. Safe.

When I came to, Dr. Siegel was counting...I heard his voice coming more into range at "six...now seven...eight..." Now closer and clearer... "Up to nine...and now at ten, opening your eyes here in my office."

Groggy.

Yawning like when a child wakes up.

Slow.

"What happened?'"

And of course, his reply: "Can you tell me?"

It would be a few more sessions before I'd come to meet the part of me that was able to open that door. This was the self-state, as Dr. Siegel would explain in one of our later sessions, that wasn't afraid to open the door. The state that could walk through the door. The state that could face being burnt. The state that also knew all along who was in there, who was chasing me on my bike.

But during that session, all I remember is being dizzy and disappearing. I knew something had happened; I just couldn't remember what.

THOUGH I WAS FEELING DISORIENTED, I knew that this, what we'd begun doing, was work I had to do. Wanted to do. Could do. I just had no idea how. When I showed up at Dr. Siegel's office for our next session, he was quiet. I sat down on the couch, immediately closed my eyes, and was afraid to speak.

I think this may have been the beginning of the period when I would arrive at his office and my tears—like the tears that had brought me to him in the first place—would begin to flow almost immediately upon sitting or lying down. No feelings, no sounds, just tears stream-ing. I couldn't stop them.

That day I was just sitting there with tears pouring out of my closed eyes, and when I finally opened them, Dr. Siegel was sitting across from me in his chair with the kindest face I had ever seen. I could see his concern, his care. I picked up the Kleenex box he had placed by my side, wiped my eyes and asked him,

"What happened last session?"

"What do you remember about it?"

"I don't remember. I mean we were talking; you were counting down...you got to eight or maybe seven, and I felt relaxed...grounded... safe, secure...and then...When I opened my eyes, it was nearly time for me to go. I felt out of it and exhausted. And I know something happened, but I have no idea what. No memory of anything after 'seven.' But all weekend I've been filled with what I assume are implicit feelings...terror...body pains...like my body is on fire...Some feelings I can't even describe to you. I can't say it...I just can't say it...something bad. It's like liquid terror is poisoning my blood and going everywhere! I just can't say what it really feels like."

"What makes it hard to say?"

"I can't say it. I don't know how to say it."

Then, after a long silence—me with eyes closed and tears still pouring—I tell him:

"I can't tell you what it felt like because you'll hate me."

His presence in the room was palpable. He spent a lot of time resonating with me before he spoke. He was attuned to me—to how much pain I was feeling, how much terror...to how hard this was. He assured me he would never hate me for anything I remembered feeling or doing. No matter what I did, remembered, or felt. It felt good to know he was there with me. I knew he meant what he said, and I felt certain he wouldn't hate me. But a part of me wasn't ready to take the chance that he might.

After another period of silence, I told him, "Please. Tell me what's happening."

He said he believed he knew what was going on with me and was ready to share his thoughts with me if I was ready to hear.

The fear of something bad about to happen popped up in my awareness...but it was quieted by his presence.

"Okay."

He told me he believed I had something known as Multiple Personality Disorder, or MPD.

Fuck. Sybil*? Surreal.*

"So, crazy after all?"

"No, Sally. Not crazy. In fact, I would say it's the exact opposite of crazy."

Tears streaming, I asked him to tell me more.

He told me that MPD was a controversial and much misunderstood diagnosis. He explained it was the result of experiencing consistent and severe abuse or neglect from a trusted caregiver before the age of seven. He called it an adaptation to being terrified and terrorized by the people a child is hardwired to depend on for safety—their parents.

"It is, Sally, a brilliant adaptation to severe abuse. When children that age are hurting, when they need protection and soothing, their brains are hardwired to go toward their parents for safety, protection, and soothing. But when the parents are themselves the source of the danger, pain, and terror, a child's brain can't make sense of that. It's a biological paradox—fear without solution—so the mind fragments."

"What does that mean about me?"

"Right now, we don't know what happened in your family. We're working together to unravel what life was like for you in that family. Why your mind had to find ways to adapt to it by creating different self-states that could keep you sane, protected from the reality of what was happening. It's a life-saving adaptation, in my opinion. What makes it difficult once you're out of that family is that you no longer need those adaptations to keep you safe. Our work now is to update your files."

"How does that explain why I have no memory?"

"You have little explicit memory because your brilliant young mind found a way to fragment off and create memory barriers between states, so no part of you had to know everything that was happening."

"Can you tell me more about that? Is it like that makes the states kind of my memory-keepers?"

"Kind of."

"And they're a good thing?"

"I believe so. Good that your mind fragmented those memories off. Yes. I believe that is a brilliant adaptation."

As shocking as this news was, I felt oddly calm. It was the first thing in a long time about my childhood that made sense. Fragmented—that was how I so often felt. Not crazy. Just the opposite of crazy. *Fear without solution.* Memory barriers between states. His explanation made sense of the things not making sense in my world. But still, in that very next moment...*Fuck.* It was a lot to take in.

"So fragmenting was the answer to fear without solution?"

"Yes."

"And the memory barriers between states are why I feel so lost sometimes and can't remember things?"

"Yes."

"So where do we go from here?"

"Our work now is to explore what happened in your childhood."

"It's so painful."

"I know, Sally. I want you to keep in mind that the pain you feel now sometimes, and as we go forward, is implicit—memories from the past. Our goal right now is for you to know them."

"And knowing them will help make them go away?"

"Knowing them is an important step in resolving them so that they won't remain painful. Knowing them will begin to dissolve the memory barriers between states. You'll be able to know what happened, but you won't feel the pain of it any longer."

"It'll be just something I know?"

"Yes."

"That I remember?"

"That's right."

"But I won't feel them anymore?"

Again, he said, "Yes."

"It does feel strange, but now that you say it—it makes sense, Dr. Siegel. It feels right. I mean, it is upsetting—yikes—*Sybil*—but I have no doubt you're right. But oh boy. I don't know..."

Tears. Quiet tears.

"Tell me."

I was feeling a little stunned. Took me a minute to find the words.

"I just don't know how I'll be able to explain this to Paul."

"What are you afraid of?"

"Not afraid—oddly, I'm not feeling afraid. I just don't know how to tell him. It makes me dizzy thinking about it. I would like to be able to talk to him about it without crying." I was feeling a little lost.

"Would you like me to talk to him about it first?"

"That would be great. If you could tell him, explain it—I think it will be easier for me to talk to him about it. I don't know how to explain it like you do."

Thank you, Dr. Siegel. Thank you so much.

DR. SIEGEL MADE AN APPOINTMENT to talk to Paul. He helped Paul understand MPD, what we were doing in therapy, and the direction of our work. Paul and I were able to talk about it—he was incredibly understanding and supportive. "I want you to continue working with him as long as you need, Sally—we'll get through this." Dr. Siegel also made a referral to a therapist he thought would be helpful to Paul during this time. I felt relieved, supported, and grateful. I think Paul did too.

DR. SIEGEL AND I RESUMED our sessions in the hallway with the doors. It was there that I would come to know the first state that helped me begin to understand what my life had been. At first, I couldn't be present. It was just too painful. I wasn't ready. And I think the state that *could* open the door was not ready for me to know what it knew. Dr. Siegel would count backward from ten, as he had earlier—and I'd be relaxed...grounded...focused—and I'd be right at the door...And then, to my surprise, the hallway would turn into a house, and there wasn't just one door, but a whole series of doors leading into different rooms, and each time I'd approach a room I'd disappear—poof. Then I'd wake up as I heard him counting forward from one.

At home I'd begun keeping a journal. Dr. Siegel suggested it as a way to process what was going on in our sessions. We talked about it also serving like a bulletin board where self-states could write to me, each other, and leave messages for him. After a few sessions of approaching the room and then disappearing, I began to see that some of the states were using the Bulletin Board.

"There're other states writing in the journal. Look..."

I showed him—the handwriting was different. Really different. Some were neat, elegant cursive, others childlike.

"I'm ready to meet the state that opened the door. See—she wants to meet me too." Her writing was very clear, neat. She had handwriting I wished I had.

In the journal she'd written a message to me, saying she knew I was afraid and thought she could help me understand some things.

"What do you think, Dr. Siegel?"

It seemed like a good idea to him too.

From his chair, I could hear him count: "Ten...eight...six...four... one..."

Under my blanket on the couch, I felt safe, but scared—a little frozen. I was beginning to have an awareness of her thoughts. "She's ready to come here, but she wants to make sure I'm ready."

"Are you ready?"

"Can I ask that state if it's okay for me to just hear what she has to say—to not go to the door yet?"

"Go ahead and ask inside if that's okay."

I turn inward...and it's not so much that I hear a voice, but I get the message that...yes, it seems like an okay idea. Then I kind of disappear, a little like a ghost who can still hear what's going on. I sit up, or she does. She opens her eyes. Sees Dr. Siegel. He greets her.

"Welcome."

"Hi."

"Thank you for coming. How are you?"

"I'm alright."

"Do you know who I am?"

"I think so."

In the silence I can hear both voices. Neither are mine. I feel invisible. I feel like I can be there but not known. It was a strange sensation.

"You're the doctor who wants to help. The one who helped me get her to the door."

"Yes. How was that for you?"

"It was good. I'm glad she got to at least get close. Thank you."

"Good for who to get close?"

"Her...you know...Sally...your patient. I wrote her the note she showed you."

"Thank you. Can you tell me your name?"

"I'm Jennifer."

"Welcome, Jennifer, so nice to meet you."

"Nice to meet you."

"Can you tell me a little about yourself?"

"What do you want to know?"

"Well, how old were you when you were born?"

"I was born when Sally was four. I was sixteen—twelve years older. Like her oldest sister."

"Okay. Can you tell me what your purpose was?"

"To keep her safe."

"Wow—that's great. How would you keep her safe?"

"By knowing things—like how dangerous things were—which she didn't—and helping her escape when she couldn't on her own. To keep her from knowing everything. I could know things she couldn't."

"Do you know everything?"

"I know a lot. What do you know?"

"I know a little. I'm finding things out as Sally does."

"Do you think it's time to share it with her?"

"How do you feel about us asking her?"

"You ask."

"Shall we ask together?"

In my ghostlike world, I could hear them both asking me if I was ready to know what was behind the door. I could hear them inviting me to join them. For the first time in a while here I heard my own voice.

"Will I be safe?"

The state called Jennifer said it was scary because it was something that happened that was not safe. Dr. Siegel assured me he would be there with me every step of the way, and he reminded me that whatever I saw or heard or felt or smelled or tasted, it was implicit...it was a memory. I was really scared...A little voice in my head kept saying "I'm 'a-scared,'" like a little child...So, I came forward and opened my eyes to see Dr. Siegel opposite me...

"It's me...Sally...I'm ready." I was scared, but ready. I felt safe with him there with me.

"Would you like to meet Jennifer first?"

"If she wants to meet me."

"Hi Sally." It was her. "It's good to see you here."

"Thank you for helping me."

Dr. Siegel did a little guided imagery, helping me visualize myself in a safe place, helping me feel protected from any harm...no matter what I saw or felt, I would be safe. It was safe for me to know whatever it was. He was there in the office with me, and Jennifer already knew what it was. No harm would come to me.

I was picturing a house again, but this time it reminded me of a house from my time in college; I'd liked the house because my friends lived there. I'd always liked hanging out there. It felt safe. I got to the front and was able to open the door. No heat. Walking in, it looked familiar—but suddenly there was a sense of real danger for me. I could hear Dr. Siegel asking me if I was okay.

"I think so."

"Would it help to share what's happening with me?"

"Yes." That felt good. "I'm in the house. It reminds me of a house in college. I liked it here, but something doesn't feel right. I'm scared."

"Is Jennifer still with you?"

"Yes."

I follow her up the big staircase. We come to a door. She tells me it's safe to open it—she lets me know it won't burn my hand. I open the door...heart in my throat with fear, closing my eyes as I step in...

"It's empty!"

I enter the room, and I see there's another door. Moving in slow motion, I go through the door...It seems like someone is leading me to the next room. Not Jennifer—it's just me. Suddenly I'm feeling afraid, and small, and vulnerable...I can't scream, and I want to...I can see in the next room...

I think tears are pouring out of my eyes. I see it...I see it...

"Sally, I'm here. How can I help you?" I hear Dr. Siegel's voice.

I want to tell him what I see. How can I tell him this? I disappear, but I can hear the little girl...*I'm a-scared...I'm a-scared...a-scared...*She is so little...and he is so big on top of her...My body is feeling it...feeling it down there...no...no...stop...it's all wet...oh no...oh no...oh no...she peed...she's gonna be in trouble for that...he's breathing hard...his face is so...so...so...red...messed up...he looks like a devil...he's screeching...huffing...puffing...she is crying...stop crying... "Don't you cry...don't you make a sound...I'll kill you if you don't shut up..." It hurts...it hurts...please stop bouncing...stop...stop...I hate this feeling...hate this feeling...I want to kill the feeling...kill my body... "That's what you get..." Something happens...oh no...oh no...I need to scream...scream... *Don't scream...he'll kill you...let me show you what to do...you can do it...it's okay...it won't hurt...let me help...there... there you go...not so bad...see...you can make it feel good...it's better like that...it's safer like that...just close your eyes...don't open your eyes...go to the tree...it's right there...you can't be hurt there...close your eyes...*

"DR. SIEGEL, I HAVE TO KNOW."

"Know what?"

My head was still spinning from our last session. Afterward I'd had a very difficult night with more awful dreams. One dream that repeated itself was me as a young girl in Galveston, waiting in the pitch-dark night for my father outside of his office, when a witch dressed all in black appeared before me and gave me a box to give my father. Opening it, I saw it had a bunch of dead kittens in it.

"Dr. Siegel"...and I knew what he was going to say before I even asked, but I asked just the same..."Seeing what I saw yesterday—that little girl being abused—was that me?"

"Tell me what you think."

"I can't figure out how it could be anyone but me—how would I feel all those things that were happening to her if it wasn't me? How could I be going through any of this if that wasn't me? I must know. I want to figure out what happened in my childhood. I have to know—"

"I think we're going to find out, Sally—I think the answers are inside. I know how hard this is."

I knew he was right. But it was really hard. After I woke up crying and visibly shaken from the dead kitten dream, Paul—alarmed by seeing me like that—had asked how therapy was going. I wasn't sure what to tell him. I honestly didn't have words. I let him know therapy was hard—the hardest thing I'd ever faced. But I knew I needed to do it.

"It's so hard, Paul. I don't know what else to say. I'm beginning to get an idea of how abusive my childhood was, and it scares me. But I must know what happened to me. It's hard to explain."

"I think I understand, Sal—I know what you and Dr. Siegel are working on is hard. I understand it's private. It's okay." I knew he understood—as much as he could. We didn't speak much about MPD. It was such a complex thing to unravel—and it had so much stigma attached to it. Mostly he was just worried for me.

"How can I help you when you wake up like this, so terrified, Sally?" he was asking me now. "Please, let me know what I can do."

"By going back to sleep if you can. I'll go downstairs until I can get back to sleep. I'll be okay."

Generally, Paul and I could talk about everything. Sometimes we didn't even need to talk—we kind of knew what the other was thinking. I was never afraid to tell him anything. But this was different. It was the beginning of a really difficult time for us both. I couldn't explain what was happening—what I was going through—I just didn't have the words. There was not much I could do except go downstairs so he could sleep. Something that would help me get centered was quietly checking on Sam, sound asleep in his room that was all cowboys, teddy bears, and soft blankets. Safe. It represented everything wonderful about childhood and being a mom to me. It was my favorite room in our house, and I loved being in it.

Being with Sam was where I felt the most grounded and safe. Safe because it was my job to keep him safe. During this time, outside of therapy, I was most focused on being Sam's mom. I was mesmerized by his joy and his remarkable development. Looking at him, and knowing about where his life had begun, gave me great hope—I could see his resilience and that gave me strength. It was a great joy Paul and I shared. It gave us both strength.

But while I was able to be present with Sam and I felt I was holding up well as his mom, it seemed like other relationships in my life were getting thrown off track. My closest friends also knew I was going through something intense in therapy. They knew it had to do with my childhood. I was also beginning to understand that talking about childhood abuse was not an easy topic for anyone. As Paul would come to say to me once, "Nothing clears a room faster, Sally, than talking about your childhood abuse." How could anyone make sense of what I was going through when I didn't understand it yet? It was difficult for everyone and everywhere. Except of course, with Dr. Siegel in his office.

I trusted him completely. And I was understanding more about MPD, both as I was living it and as Dr. Siegel was teaching me about it, always explaining it in the most positive terms. I was learning from him and reading books about MPD as I experienced it—in my dreams, in my memory lapses, in the Bulletin Board and within the safety of therapy. It was intense and often overwhelming. But I was determined to figure out what had happened. Something was the cause of the things I was experiencing. I needed to know what.

SINCE THE I-HOPE-IT'S-NOT-MOM CALL with my oldest sister, we hadn't spoken. I was curious if she'd shared our conversation with anyone. I imagined not, as I was understanding more and more about how no one in my family spoke about much of anything. Still, had she said anything to them? I just didn't know. What I did know was I wanted some answers. To do that, I decided to visit my parents. I was a little nervous to tell Dr. Siegel.

When I told him what I was thinking, he asked me to tell him more.

"I just need to be with them. To see them. To find out how I feel with them. I need to know what it feels like to be in their presence now that I'm doing all this work."

He said he thought it might be a good idea, but he also wanted to make sure I felt safe. He was relieved when I told him a girlfriend I'd gone to high school and college with, Susan, lived near my parents and would accompany me on my visit. And I'd be staying at a hotel, not with them. I was also taking Sam because I hadn't yet left him overnight and I thought it'd be best if he came with me. I'd also scheduled the trip pretty deliberately: I would be going over the weekend, back on Sunday, and I could see Dr. Siegel as planned that Monday. Perfect. As I prepared to leave his office, he asked me how I was feeling about going. "Good," I said. Then I just sat there for a few minutes, and I felt my tears begin to flow. These tears did not feel so much like tears of fear. More like trepidation. I had no idea what would happen. I'd also come to understand tears weren't always about fear or even sadness. Sometimes they were simply energy moving through my body. Emotions. Always a release. Knowing that, I could welcome them.

As I got up to go, Dr. Siegel asked me what I was thinking.

"I'm thinking, Dr. Siegel, that I've just begun to scratch the surface. I have no expectations for this visit except to maybe know more than I know now." But I had no idea at all what that would be.

Oddly I did not feel the terror at that moment, thinking about seeing them. I just knew I had to go.

PAUL TOOK SAM AND ME TO LAX to catch our flight. I'm not sure Paul understood why I was going. But he was supportive of my therapeutic work. It helped him knowing that Dr. Siegel and I had discussed it.

When we arrived, I checked into the hotel and waited for Susan. She was a great friend. I'd known her since I was fifteen, when my family moved to Galveston from Chapel Hill. She had lived down the street from me there and spent time with my family. We'd gone to the same high school and college and never lost touch. I was so happy she had agreed to meet me for this visit. Once she arrived, I realized I wasn't ready to see my parents—I felt a little sick to my stomach at the thought. It had been a little over a year since I'd seen them, but I hadn't been in therapy then, so I had no idea what it would be like seeing them now. I called and told them we would come in the morning. Talking about it all with Susan over dinner that night was good. When we'd spoken on the phone, I'd filled her in about the work I was doing with Dr. Siegel. Now, I asked her to tell me her memories about what I was like and what my family was like when she'd known me in high school. She told me that she had always been afraid of my dad. That her dad thought my dad was, in his words, a son-of-a-bitch.

What she said about my mom was, "Well, of course I remember she was always drunk."

"Drunk?" I was stunned.

She couldn't believe this was news to me.

"Sally—she almost killed us a couple times driving. Yes—she was always drunk!"

Always?

I did remember my oldest sister once saying, when I was in my twenties, how hard Mom's drinking had been for her growing up. I'd had no memory of her drinking, of course, but my sister was twelve years older, so I guess I'd figured Mom had stopped drinking by the time I was born. Which apparently was not remotely the case, if what Susan was saying was true.

By now it was really sinking in how fucked up it was that I had no memory of my parents. I was grateful for friends like Susan who did, and I was even more curious now to see how I would feel when I went to see them the next morning.

I slept well that night. I felt safe with one of my best friends and memory keeper, and of course Sam. There was, however, a surreal sense to it all. Was I floating? Ghosting? Who was I? I was becoming more and more confused...and more and more curious but cautious.

IT WAS A VERY BRIEF VISIT.

On the plane home, I was really shaken. In the time I'd spent with my parents, I'd had a glimpse of something that was at once horrifying and enlightening. It was the first time I'd gotten the feeling of something awful about to happen—and been able to act on it. In my sessions with Dr. Siegel, I'd recognized the fear we were uncovering was implicit; I'd also often had a strong awareness that there was a danger driving the fear, even if I didn't know exactly what that danger was. But this time, I'd known exactly who was in danger. Sam. I had to protect Sam. It was primal. Now, sitting in my seat aboard the plane, with little Sammy next to me sleeping soundly—my baby, my son. Loved. Cared for. Known. Understood. Protected. Seen. Joy-filled. I closed my eyes, and all I could picture was the moment I'd seen her taking his tiny hand...

"What are you doing, Mom?"

'Taking him to the bathroom."

"Why?" (Not *Why are you doing that, you crazy bitch?*, which is what I'd been thinking.)

"He's fidgety...he needs to go to the bathroom."

Every instinct in me said *no*. I quickly went over to take Sam's hand in mine and keep him close to me.

"He doesn't need to go to the bathroom, Mom, he's in a diaper."

And her face fell, looked different, not like any image I recalled... but it kind of reminded me of something.

"He's still in a diaper? Sally, he's too big to be in a diaper."

No mom, he's not too big. He's little. A little boy. He's still in a diaper.

I felt sick to my stomach.

"Do you have extra diapers with you?"

I do. I absolutely do. I'm a mom, Mom. I'm a good mom. I take care of my child. What the fuck is this? He's a little kid. I always have a diaper— right here—in my diaper bag. You stupid fucking freak. An anger I wasn't familiar with had welled up within. I didn't need to scream. I didn't need to say a thing. I was feeling that fight/flight/freeze response that, Dr. Siegel had explained to me, happens when our brainstem sends a signal of threat. We become aware of danger. Quickly assess for danger. Then choose our action of defense: stay and fight, flee to safety, or freeze our body because there are no other choices. Right now, though, I wasn't in a panic, nor was I freezing. Quite the contrary. I knew what I had to do—stand up for my son—and I was doing it. Felt strength from within. What a feeling that was.

"Well, why don't you and Susan leave him here, and I'll watch him while you go shopping—spend some time together."

The feeling was dreamlike—it felt as if I was straddling two worlds again. Me, my son, my mother, and him...all in this room...I saw a green blanket on the bed...felt a sensation...creepy...Looking at her, I felt my whole body go numb, which was the strangest sensation. And there was a smell. A smell that made me want to vomit.

I had to get out of there. Fast.

"You know, I think we're going back to the hotel—I feel a little sick— I'll call later."

I picked up Sam. Grabbed my diaper bag, got Susan to drive us back to the hotel. Then I called the airline and booked us on the next flight home that afternoon. Susan was upset to see me so upset, but she understood—again, as much as anyone could.

I was out of there.

And now, on the flight home, sitting with my wonderful boy safely next to me, I was filled with feelings. Implicit. Memories of feelings. Flashes of her. The green blanket. Hurt. Full-body pain. Shaky but safe, now. Thinking also of my oldest sister's voice...

...and her words...

"I hope it's not Mom."

For the first time in my life, I found it necessary to have the air sickness bag on a plane ready to use.

PAUL PICKED US UP from the airport and could see how shaken I was. I didn't tell him everything that happened—I couldn't explain anything that happened—but I was feeling how upsetting it all was. Visibly upset, mad and angry. Even as I felt loving, too, with Sam and Paul now. It may have been the first time I had an awareness of the *internal* feeling of switching, outside of Dr. Siegel's office—of the experience of different states swirling; of trying to figure things out. Feeling a little lost.

When we got home and Sam was asleep, I reflected with Paul on what had happened as best I could—why we left so abruptly.

"You know, Sally, your parents have always been bit of a quandary to me."

We'd never talked much about my parents—which was odd, since Paul's family was such a big part of our lives. It was a relief to hear he'd found them confusing. When I asked him to explain just what he meant, he said they just never seemed to match up to how I had portrayed them. It was clear he never liked them much. He'd found them troubling long before I had. I was beginning to see them more clearly only now. Like so many other things, I just couldn't understand how I simply hadn't registered any of the things about my parents that others saw so clearly. But then I could hear Dr. Siegel describing

MPD—a lifesaving protective measure for a young child growing up in unspeakable circumstances where survival depended on *not* knowing.

"You couldn't know, Sally," he'd told me. "You were just a baby! A little girl. It wasn't knowable. Thank goodness your mind fragmented. It saved you."

And that fragmentation had persisted, even after I was no longer a child. But now I was beginning to know what, in the past, couldn't be known. It felt like my brain was going through a process of reconfiguration. Updating files. Certain parts of my body and mind thawing. Sometimes it felt like I could feel my brain shifting. Yet I still didn't have answers...Who was that little girl and who was hurting her? I mean, I was coming to know some things. But I felt I needed to really know the *whole* thing. I wanted the truth.

I did *know* it had to do with them—with my parents. The feelings I'd felt in the past, visiting them—the feelings of being completely frozen at night and not sleeping because I might be killed—had flooded my senses this visit, when I was there with Sam. Before I could never quite figure out where the feelings came from—was I just crazy?—but now I knew, the feelings came from them. Something about them being my parents—what they'd done or were capable of doing. I could feel it all. The feeling of fear without solution. That was the feeling of being in the room with them. The fear was there. Now to figure out exactly why...

But the fear was there. That I couldn't deny.

The fear was of them.

EVENTUALLY PAUL AND I WENT TO BED and fell asleep. I slept a little but was awakened by this full-body feeling of something happening to me—something awful. Horrible feelings...crazy feelings...laying there in bed next to Paul, who was sound asleep—yes—frozen with fear—I couldn't move. I was remembering visiting my parents' house this one time before Paul and I were married...I could remember clearly feeling as if I was being sexually assaulted...Not a memory of someone attacking me...not a visual awareness of being raped...but a feeling of being sexually aroused just by being in the house...that house...their house...like it was happening in front of everyone and I just had to pretend it wasn't happening. What the fuck...it was bizarre...paralyzed me...I knew it was so crazy. I knew nothing was happening, and I felt powerless...I felt trapped...It was terrifying, demoralizing, and *shameful*. What was going on? I had no idea...

Then Paul woke up... "What's going on, Sally...What's wrong?"

"I don't know..." I wasn't crying, but I was kind of in shock, I think. It felt shocking.

I think it may have been the first time Paul had gotten a real sense of what was happening to me. MPD—abusive childhood...He'd told Dr. Siegel when they met that he'd never noticed any abrupt shifts in my state of mind. "Nothing out of the ordinary, doctor—just what I think of as normal mood swings..." Now he was seeing how upsetting it had been for me to see my parents. And I could see it too. Feel it. Paul just hugged me.

"It'll be okay, Sally. You're home now."

Being there with Paul—Sam asleep in his room across the hall, I felt so safe...and not just because I was home—but because I'd made it out of my parents' house alive.

"I never want to see or speak to them again," I told Paul.

He hugged me even closer and said, "You never have to."

I never did.

As I was closing my eyes, hoping to get back to sleep, all I could see was her taking Sam's tiny hand, and the green blanket that'd been on the bed, and I felt sick all over again. I put my pillow over my face immediately and I felt light, as if I might be leaving my body. I worked hard to stay where I was. They weren't the parents I had believed them to be. Portrayed or pretended them to be. Perhaps wished them to be. It was like I'd come to know this for the first time. And I was more determined than ever to dig deeper. The dreams, the sessions I couldn't be present for—the answers to all this were buried in my childhood. And who was in charge of my childhood? Them. My fucking parents. The people who were supposed to care for me. And even though I had no explicit memories of childhood, I was filled with implicit ones, all of them horrible. I couldn't conjure up one good memory of either of them. I was so happy to be seeing Dr. Siegel in the morning to talk about it.

DRIVING IN FOR MY APPOINTMENT the next morning, I was still feeling sick to my stomach. And even though it felt like I might throw up, I really needed to get to therapy to talk to Dr. Siegel about it all. I knew talking to him would help.

When I walked into his office, I think he could tell I wasn't feeling so great.

"What's going on, Sally?"

I told him about leaving my parents' early...about what'd happened that night I got home—about the awful feelings.

"It didn't feel like a nightmare, Dr. Siegel...I was completely awake. I just don't know what it was. It was horrible...horrible feelings."

He took his time, as he often did, and then said, "Sounds like you may have been having a flashback, Sally."

The only thing I knew about flashbacks was they happened to war vets believing they were in the middle of battle when actually they were safely home. I asked him to explain more.

"A flashback, Sally, is when, as you are recalling a traumatic event, you actually reexperience it as if you are still in it—as if it's happening now—there is no feeling of it coming from your past."

"Like implicit memories?"

"Yes. Remember, implicit memory is likely involved in flashbacks."

His explanation made sense, even if it didn't make the flashback better, but at least I knew more.

"So, not crazy."

"No Sally, not crazy. Those were feelings from a long time ago."

"Seeing my parents made them come up?"

"I think so."

I went from sitting in the chair across from him to laying down on the couch. I was exhausted from it all. I brought him up to date on what had transpired at my parents and how Paul had helped me with the flashback.

We both were quiet for a while. Then he asked me what I was thinking about.

I let him know I was ready to continue our work unraveling my childhood. "I have some answers to that question now," I said.

"What question?"

"When you asked me for adjectives describing my relationship with my mother."

"Wow. Please do tell me."

I hadn't thought of the words until just this moment. I'd known they were there. I'd felt them. But until this moment I hadn't heard them; I hadn't been able to unearth them and say them to myself. Lying on Dr. Siegel's couch, I could still feel the danger I felt with my parents. Now I thought I might have the words to actually describe that danger to him.

"Stuck. Or not 'stuck'—no, it was the feeling of not being able to move."

That wasn't exactly the feeling either. I was having trouble finding the right word. I felt the feeling. I knew the feeling. I couldn't think what to call it.

"Trapped...like I couldn't get out of there. Like I just couldn't do anything."

That's still not exactly it.

"It feels a little like—like I just can't go anywhere. I have to stay. I can't move..."

Dr. Siegel was listening so closely.

"Being there—being with them and having Sam and Susan with me—I felt frightened."

My voice said "frightened," but in my head I heard "a-scared," like the little girl from before.

A scared little girl.

A-scared.

It hit me.

"Oh god."

"What, Sally?"

"I think it's the feeling of being a little kid."

"Can you stay with the feeling of being a little kid and see what comes up?"

"I'm feeling sick to my stomach."

"Do you need help?"

"No. It's all right. I felt it almost the minute we landed there. On the flight home I was hanging on to the bag they give you."

"The air sickness bag?"

"Yes."

"Did you ever throw up?"

"No—but the feeling won't go away."

Mind racing.

"Stay with the feeling if you can."

"You know, I wasn't frightened there for me, really—I just got flooded with those feelings—I knew I was okay. From the moment I walked in there with Sam and Susan, I felt flooded with...like I was in slow motion there. And then...and then...oh god...this huge alarm bell went off in my head...for Sam."

I told him about when she took his hand...I had to close and scrunch my eyes up so tight even to say it. I could see it...I could see it...

"What could you see, Sally?"

"The green blanket."

It took my breath away. I was very quiet. I started to cry.

And shake.

Everything was in slow motion. Slow motion.

"The feelings were so large, Dr. Siegel. It was big and scary...so frightened for Sam."

I opened my eyes.

"I was out of there."

I felt like I had to keep talking about what happened—how it felt like slow motion...how she just was giving me the creeps...the green blanket...Sam's tiny hand...I just had to get Sam away from her. Away from there. I felt like I was able to stay present, but there were flickers of me not being fully there. The slow-motion thing.

"I kept smelling something. Something that made me feel sick to my stomach. I needed to get out of there fast. I was afraid I would throw up."

We were quiet for a while.

"How did it feel to be able to protect Sam?"

"Powerful. Safe. I felt safe keeping him safe."

I just sat there going over and over it in my mind.

"Keeping Sam safe mobilized me! That was the feeling! That was it. I felt completely immobilized until I had to take care of him. It was so strange. Like if I moved I would...I don't know...it would hurt if I moved an inch. There was an awareness that being in that place with them was not safe for...oh my god..."

Tears flowing...body shaking...crying, sobbing, not just tears...

"What's going on, Sally?"

"It's not safe for little kids."

We sat there for a few minutes. Eyes closed. More tears. Quiet tears, now, replacing the crying-out-loud kind. He handed me the Kleenex box. I was just sitting there silent, crying. After some more time he asked me,

"Do you know the meaning of the green blanket?"

"I don't know exactly. I think, though, it's when I started to feel sick to my stomach."

"When you saw it?"

"Yes."

"Would it help to ask inside if there is a state that knows about it?"

"I think so."

I got more comfortable on the couch. Even as I did that, prepared myself to go inward, I wasn't sure if I could take any more in just yet.

"I feel sick...I'm not sure I can do this."

"Can you let that feeling come into awareness?"

I was getting the creepiest feelings, and the green blanket was flashing in my mind. It was making my body jolt...as if the flashes of memory were assaulting me and my whole body was reacting.

"Can you tell me what the creepiest feelings are?"

"I think something bad is going to happen. Or that I'm about to see something I don't want to see."

I was crying more and more. Slow motion. And I shuddered in fear. Like my body was having a seizure of some kind.

"What's that, Sally?"

"Having Sam with me got me out of there. Having Susan felt like back-up. Dr. Siegel, I don't know what would've happened if I'd been there alone."

"Would it help to ask for help inside?"

"I think so."

"Remember Sally, you can use the remote control."

Earlier in therapy, especially when I'd been exploring the hallway of doors with memories, Dr. Siegel helped me devise a system where I could imagine sitting in a screening room of sorts in which I could watch any video I needed to. I alone had access to the videos, and to a remote control, so I could start and stop any memory whenever I needed to.

"You're in charge, Sally, of stopping and starting it."

"Okay." I took a breath to steady myself. "I need a part to help me with this."

"Can you ask inside for that help?"

Sitting there with so much fear, I couldn't even ask for help.

"Dr. Siegel?"

"Yes?"

"Could you ask for me?"

"Do you want me to help you ask or ask for you?"

"Together."

Dr. Siegel would speak, we decided. My invitation would be internal.

"I'd like to invite any state that would like to help Sally with this memory that is coming up for her."

"Thank you," I told Dr. Siegel.

"You're welcome."

That now-familiar deep dive inside. Body feeling slow. Sleepy. I could feel my eyes flutter...rolling up in my head...long, long silence. Holding the remote ready to push stop if I needed to...It would always take a while for something to emerge as I went inside, but slowly eyes opened—a little...as if coming out of hiding. I felt a jolt...my body quietly shaking now...

I'm diving deeper inside.

Long silence. I can hear the silence. Not completely gone.

"Hi."

I could hear a faint, tiny voice. Child-like. Scared. *A-scared.*

"Hello there." I could hear Dr. Siegel welcoming the tiny voice.

The state nods its head as if to say thank you. I get the feeling it's not so much afraid to speak as that it's not practiced at speaking. Doesn't have the words. And then again, Dr. Siegel's voice,

"Can I ask you something?"

"Uh-huh."

"Do you have a name?"

Nods again.

"Can you tell me your name?"

"Little Sally."

"Welcome, Little Sally. Thank you for coming. Do you know if Sally is listening?"

"She is. Jennifer too."

"Do you know who I am?"

"I think so."

"I'm Dr. Siegel."

"You're helping Sally."

"Yes."

"Thank you."

"Oh, you're so welcome. Okay. I want to remind Sally that if she needs to, she can press stop with the remote control."

"She says okay."

"Can you tell me when you were born?"

"When I was really little."

"Before five?"

"I think so. Maybe around three. When the other one started kindergarten."

"Who is the other one?"

"The one that's two years older."

"Another state?"

"No—the sister."

"Oh, the sister who's two years older?"

Nods yes.

"Okay. Thanks for that. Can you share with me what your purpose was?"

"I'm too little to know."

"Can you tell me too little to know what?"

"Just too little to know. Sally wants to say something to you."

"Okay. Can Sally come talk?"

"It's me."

"Sally?"

"Yes. I feel sick, Dr. Siegel."

"Can you tell me what is going on?"

"Something about Little Sally and the green blanket and my mother."

"Do you need to push the hold button?"

"I think I can stay. I want to stay. I don't think Little Sally can stay. She's too little."

"Okay Sally. Thank you, Little Sally."

"I think she's sleeping. She says goodbye."

It was so dark, and the smell was so strong.

"She's just lying there—like she's dead."

"Little Sally is dead?"

"No, my mother. Little Sally is right by her. On the green blanket. There's vomit all over the blanket. There's vomit on Little Sally. I feel sick. I'm going to push stop. It's making me sick. I think Jennifer wants to come to help."

"Okay, Sally. I'm going to put the trash can by you if you need to be sick."

"I don't think she's going to be sick. It just feels like it."

"Is that Jennifer?"

"Yes."

"Hi. Welcome—thank you for coming again."

"I think I can help Sally understand what is happening," Jennifer says.

"Shall we make sure she's ready to hear?"

"She's listening."

"Okay."

"You know how Sally told you she felt sick when she saw her parents?"

"Yes."

"You see—Sally is only just learning—kind of putting some pieces of memory together that her mom was always drunk. Her mom was a drunk. Like her friend Susan told her...All the time. And what makes her feel sick to her stomach is the smell of bourbon."

"The smell of bourbon on her mother's breath?"

"And in her vomit."

"Oh, I see."

"As for Little Sally, she thinks her mom is dead."

"Can you explain a little more about that?"

"Her mom was always drunk. Little Sally would be home alone with her a lot, once her two-years-older sister was in kindergarten. So Little Sally would just lie there with her mom, afraid she was dead. And she would try to make her not dead."

"How would she try to make her mom not dead?"

"I can't talk about that now."

"Can you tell me why you can't talk about it now?"

"It's the creepy feeling."

"I see."

"There's a lot of stuff about the green blanket, Dr. Siegel. I can't talk about it now."

"Can you tell me why?"

"I don't think Sally is ready to know. She wants to push the stop button. We can't see any more now. Little Sally and other little parts spent a lot of time on the green blanket."

"Thank you, Jennifer. It's so helpful."

"I want to tell you one more thing. Sally can hear too."

"What's that?"

"The smell is what her mother throws up on the blanket. And Little Sally has to clean it up."

"The smell of bourbon?"

"Yes."

"How would she have to clean it up?"

I immediately pressed the stop button and nearly jumped off the couch sitting up.

"I can't know this, Dr. Siegel."

"All right," he said, sitting back in his chair. His eyes, as always, were kind. "You're always in charge, Sally."

I was kind of in shock.

"Something about the green blanket. Feeling sick. Feeling other things too."

"What other things?"

"I can't say it." The words came out in a rush. "I can't know it. I can't tell you."

"Okay. It's okay, Sally. Would you like to stop now?"

"Okay."

"Shall we say goodbye for now to Jennifer?"

"She wants to say one thing."

"Is it okay with you?"

I wanted to check in with Jennifer to make sure she only talked about the one thing. The smell thing. Not the other feeling thing.

"Yes."

Jennifer explained to Dr. Siegel that when Little Sally would do things to try and wake her mother up, which for Little Sally meant she wasn't dead anymore, her mother would be furious about the vomit that smelled like bourbon. She would make Little Sally clean it up. Little Sally was too little to do that very well and she didn't know how to clean things so she would try to put it in her mouth. And that would make her vomit sometimes and her mother would spank her really hard. With a long ruler. It hurt. Really bad.

At the end of the session, I couldn't speak. Or open my eyes. I knew what had happened. It was horrible to hear. But it was beginning to make sense. Horrible sense.

I could barely speak.

"What are you thinking, Sally?"

"I don't know how to think about this, Dr. Siegel. I mean...I'm starting to understand why I never remembered things. It's so horrible."

I could feel the sting of being hit with the ruler on my body.

I was quiet again for a while. Thinking. Not thinking. Feeling. Not feeling. Knowing. Not knowing. Poor Little Sally.

"Little Sally is me."

"How are you thinking about that?"

"I'm not sure. I mean...crazy...what makes sense is crazy."

"Remember, you're not crazy."

"I know. I guess what I'm thinking most now is not that *I'm* crazy. It's that they were."

"Crazy?"

"Yes."

"What's that like for you to think about?"

"I don't know yet, Dr. Siegel."

I just didn't know.

As I was leaving that day, I had flashes of the green blanket and of my mother screaming at me.

Clean it up.

Go ahead. Now.

And don't you dare throw that up.

"Are you still feeling sick to your stomach?" Dr. Siegel had asked, just before I walked out the door.

No. No, I wasn't. Not sick to my stomach. I was feeling sick all over. And the other feelings were invading me.

A FEW DAYS LATER, I got a call from my oldest sister. We'd gone from speaking often, pre-therapy, to barely speaking now. I hardly thought of her, or any of my siblings. They just weren't in my thoughts at all. I never wondered whether I was the only one anything had happened to. They were all, with the exception of the only-two-years-older sister, a decade or more older than me. Did they know? What was it like for them? I had no idea.

My sister had heard from our mother.

"Yeah—she's upset because she said you just disappeared."

"Yes, I decided to leave early."

"What's going on?"

What to say? I could hear Dr. Siegel's voice telling me, *the truth is your friend.* I decided to go with that...as best I could.

"You know, I'm in therapy right now. And I'm remembering things about my childhood."

I was curious what she'd say...was she curious?

"What have you found out?"

The truth is your friend. Maybe.

"I'm doing a lot of work figuring this all out. I'm fine sharing it with you, but I don't need to. And—it's not good. So, don't ask if you aren't able to hear the truth."

"Please tell me."

"I think they were horrible to me. Abusive. Awful. Scary. Mostly I'm having memories of being terrified of them. I left early because I was afraid for Sam to be near them."

"Not just Dad?"

"No. Not just him."

Until she said it, I hadn't even thought about how little he'd played into how I was feeling that day at their place.

There was a bit of a pause.

"Well, in a way that helps explain some things I never really understood before."

Wow. I hadn't been expecting that. Like what? What did it explain?

"Mom's said things to me, over the years, about not understanding why you're so nice to her...that she knew she'd done some awful things to you. I never understood that. Especially things when you were little."

"What things?"

"She never told me what."

I imagined that meant my sister had never asked.

"Well, I'm working on it. I appreciate your understanding."

"Will you keep me up to date as you find out more?"

I told her I would. I was certain I wouldn't tell her the MPD part—that there were multiple different states that held on to different things. That felt very private to me still. Only Paul knew. I was glad she responded as she did. She'd seemed to understand well enough; she seemed ready to know more. Maybe? Yet I didn't feel as close to her as I used to. Everything was changing.

Boy oh boy, were things changing.

Later that same evening, I got another call from her. It was crazy. When I mentioned our earlier conversation, she denied we'd spoken, denied saying everything she'd told me. "I never said Mom said that" she said, firmly and absolutely. "You're a liar." I think she actually *believed* we hadn't spoken.

IN THAT MOMENT I DIDN'T THINK MUCH about what this might mean about her. I was caught off-guard mostly because as shocking as it was, her total denial of our original conversation also felt familiar. I'm not sure if I thought this exactly at that moment, but I'd soon come to be intensely aware of that feeling, the feeling of having lived in a world full of denial. Secrets. It was a feeling I knew—I was experiencing painful flashes of myself as a little girl with my head spinning, trying to keep up with what was what and who was who and what was happening to me. It was eerily familiar. As if from afar, I could see the confusion and despair on her face. *My* face. My face as a child.

Paul was right. My family was not how I had portrayed them. They were monsters.

Later still that night, I began to hear from my other siblings. Yelling at me: how dare I accuse their parents of abuse. One of my brothers—who'd served in the military—said he'd fought in Vietnam and knew all about abuse, "You know nothing about abuse," he screamed at me. "You're just a spoiled brat."

"I hope you drown in that ocean!"

He wanted me to drown.

Accidental hangings.

Another went on and on about how in his job he had a high-level security clearance, and he'd know if there had been abuse. One of their spouses called to assure me she'd been around when I was little, and she would've known if there had ever been abuse. And one of my siblings called to tell me she heard I was saying that—her words exactly—"Dad had fucked you as a child." How dare I say that.

That same one told me in the same breath that sure, she did remember once when Mom walked in on her when she was about seven masturbating and said:

"Feels good, doesn't it?"—and closed the door.

It was chilling.

The next day, my oldest sister's daughter—my niece—who was in high school, called me. She let me know that she'd been in the room when I initially spoke to her mom about what I was working on in therapy.

"When Mom got off the phone with you, she told me you'd said that your parents were abusive. And she told me that she did remember coming home sometimes to find her mother passed out on the floor with a bottle of whiskey and a bottle of pills."

My niece went on to say the next day she'd checked in on her mom to see how she was feeling about all this, and her mom asked her what she was talking about.

"About what Aunt Sally told you yesterday."

"I don't know what you're talking about," her mother had said.

"That you remembered your mom being passed out drunk on the floor."

"I never said that. My mom drank, but she didn't have a drinking problem."

"Mom—that's denial."

"It's not denial if it never happened."

Eventually it would surface that my mother had abused my niece as well.

When she told her mother, her mother replied,

"That wasn't my experience."

And that was that.

OVER THE NEXT COUPLE OF WEEKS, I received a series of letters and unsigned cards, all of them venomous. Some of the cards were from a greeting card series featuring a little boy and girl dressed in vintage grown-up clothes, all in sepia tones, holding hands. The cards looked sentimental, but the handwritten sentiments inside were dire and hate-filled. There was a gothic religious tone to some of them—fire and brimstone stuff. There were no death threats, but the writer, whoever it was, told me they wished I'd die. The cards were upsetting to receive—but I didn't feel afraid of them. It was kind of like for the first time, I really knew my family—even as at the same time it felt like, somewhere within, I always had. My childhood was beginning to make itself known to me.

Over the years that followed, I had occasional calls from my parents. The moment I answered the phone and heard their voices—this was in the days before caller ID—I would begin to tremble, and then I'd immediately hang up. It could take me hours to calm the feeling of terror streaming through my system after one of those calls. Implicit terror.

Eventually the letters stopped. And the calls. In the end, I didn't communicate with any of them—not my parents, and not my siblings— nor did any of the siblings attempt to reach me, for well over ten years.

DR. SIEGEL AND I SPENT MANY SESSIONS processing all this family activity. Out of everything that came up for me in the year we'd been working together, my siblings' behavior was the one thing that seemed to be making sense to me. He asked me to tell him more about that.

"I'm not sure, Dr. Siegel. It's not that I remember any of them being mean when I was little. If you asked me to give you words to describe my relationship with most of them now, though, I would say 'mean'— but I couldn't give you examples of them *being* mean. Besides the calls I've been getting now, that is. It's been more like a feeling. A feeling of disconnection. A feeling of despair. And the creepy feeling. A feeling of not being safe—of not being protected. The vulnerability of a little girl in a house full of big people with nowhere to hide. To disappear. To be invisible. Not being cared for. *Not being cared about.*"

I paused to think for a moment.

"This is all shocking, yet I'm not shocked. That's kind of the thing— shocked but not really. I have all the feelings of memory, but no memory of memory. Uncomfortable feelings. It's so confusing, and yet it feels—and I can't think of a better word—normal. Normal for them."

For so long, normal for me.

Things were changing.

And then suddenly I laughed out loud.

"What's that laugh about?"

I think I must've just sat there for a minute or two shaking my head.

"Thinking that nearly a year ago when I first came to you, and you asked me to tell you about my childhood and I said I had a good childhood. How crazy is that?"

"Not crazy."

"I know."

Sitting there, not sure what I was feeling or thinking.

"What are you feeling?

"I don't know...blank. I feel blank. I don't have easy answers for how I feel. It takes time for me to figure out what I'm feeling these days. Even when I can't feel anything at all, it takes time for me to know that."

Screaming inside.

"Would it help to take some breaths, Sally? Even close your eyes and look inward...ask inside what you're feeling?"

That's what had come to always work. And yet—at times I felt the weight of the task, how much it often took.

"For my whole life, Dr. Siegel, I can see how I've had to work so hard to keep all my feelings away from me. I guess it's going to take time now to find them again. What did you call it—mental gymnastics?"

Yes—backflips and somersaults and balance beams. The mental gymnastics of my not-crazy mind. Cartwheels.

"It's exhausting."

"We can go as slow as you want. As slow as you need."

I closed my eyes. It felt like I could descend deep inside or travel way up high to discover what feeling was. Which feeling? How do feelings feel? Where's that feeling? Where could it be hiding? I wondered where it was. Finding it was an excruciating, crushing, journey. A path I had to find and follow. And of course, I had to leave myself a trail. Breadcrumbs so I could find my way back. But if I tried...there it is. There it is. Yes. Of course. I know that feeling—there it was—not the feeling I was looking for, but a sensation, like electric currents jetting through my body, that scrambled to cut off each and every feeling before I could feel it.

It took so much energy and effort not to feel the current. I always had to feel it first before not feeling it. There was no help. There was always hurt. And the minute I knew that, the minute I felt that—*poof*—it was gone. I knew I had to find a way now, though, to feel it—the thing the current was meant to protect me from. I had to remind myself: *it's implicit*, these feelings that could feel so terrifying to me to explore. *It's a* memory *of a feeling. It's the* memory *of pain.* Working on not disappearing now...

"If you asked me right now what my childhood was like—the family I grew up in—I'd say painful. But I still couldn't tell you exactly why. What happened that created this terror and pain...It feels, Dr. Siegel, that I don't know any of them. That none of them are as I thought they were. But also, it finally makes sense. I was always confused by them. Now I know. Thing is—I really don't feel anything for them but anger."

"Your siblings?"

"Yes. I feel like I should feel sad that they have cut me out. But I don't. I feel kind of angry." And it was true—the feelings I was experiencing were *kind of* anger, and kind of something else. "But mostly..."

...on the feeling trail...mostly what?...oh yes...there it is....

"Mostly I feel relief. Why do you think that is?"

"You tell me."

"I don't miss any of them. Not even my oldest sister."

"It might be because you don't miss what you never had."

We sat there together in silence for some time. This would happen often—sometimes I just didn't have the words. I would sit with the pain, and Dr. Siegel would be right there with me. Sitting by me, every step of the way. Guiding me safely through the pain. I was afraid sometimes that my pain would hurt him, and today I told him so.

"It doesn't hurt me, Sally. I can see your pain and I understand it. I'm sorry I couldn't be there for you then."

"Thank you."

Tears flooding out of me.

"Can you tell me what you're thinking, Sally?"

"I'm thinking that I don't know them—not because of them, but because of me."

"What do you mean?"

"That they've always been the way they are. It's me that's changing. I'm feeling dizzy."

Spinning...

"Why don't you lie down on the couch, Sally."

"Okay."

...less dizzy.

"What's going on?"

"I have this awareness that there are a bunch of different ways of being with all of them."

"The siblings?"

"The whole family."

"Can you say more about that?"

Breathing deep.

"I think there is some kind of battle taking place inside of me. That there are a bunch of different states ready to say something and then a bunch that don't want any state to say anything."

The dizziness was easing. My internal vision was blurry though—like a dust storm working its way into a tornado.

"Sometimes it feels okay and then I get really upset and afraid. Like I'm going to be in trouble. Dr. Siegel..."

"What, Sally?"

"...there seems to be an awful lot of states."

"That's some big awareness."

It was. Gymnastics. Off balance. Dizzy.

"Can you tell me a little more about the feeling of being in trouble?"

"With this new awareness about my family, I feel like a ghost walking around myself. It's hard to find the words to tell you. I don't have words for what I know now. Even though I know it. It feels like—maybe something bad is going to happen."

"Can you ask inside?"

Deep within there was an awareness of many different states of mind letting me know what was ahead. At once an invitation and a warning...I could feel their presence within. I knew there was a bunch of them, but I didn't yet know any of them or their stories—except for Little Sally and Jennifer. There were more. I could feel more were coming. And I had the sensation that they were feeling so many different things. Dizzy. At one point it occurred to me that *they* might not all even know about *me*. Whatever "me" means anymore. I could feel a rumbling sensation from the inside out.

"It feels like my body needs to brace for what's to come."

"Does it feel unsafe?"

Digging even deeper inside, I asked if it was unsafe.

"I don't know...I'm not sure..."

...a long pause going deep inside to find—if not an answer, at least some information...and then...

"Maybe..."

"Maybe what?"

"Maybe not so safe."

With this Dr. Siegel sounded a little alarmed—calm yet alarmed, or at least cautious about how to proceed.

"Okay—I would like for any states that are listening to agree now that no harm will come to Sally—here in the office or when Sally goes home later."

I wasn't feeling out of my body—it was more like I was completely in my body, but it had a mind that had divided and fragmented, and that the states were all real, all me. I couldn't tell where I fit. Or how I fit. Even if. I didn't feel frozen, but I couldn't speak or move. I felt like they were all swimming inside of me. Some like dolphins. Some in a whirlpool of danger. Some could surf. Others were being pounded by the waves. Some pulled dangerously by the undertow. Some were floating. A few were drowning. And there were those gasping for air at the surface.

No more mental gymnastics. More like mental tsunami.

Dr. Siegel wanted to know if any state had heard him...

"I would like to talk to a state about safety."

I nodded.

"Can you tell me what state you are?"

And in a voice I did not know I could hear,

"It's Allison."

"Hello, Allison."

"Hello."

"Thank you for speaking up."

"You're welcome."

"Do you know who I am?"

"Yes—Dr. Siegel—thank you for helping us."

"You're welcome. First, can you tell me how old you were when you were born?"

"I was eleven—but I act older. Everyone thinks I'm older."

"How was that helpful—to be older?"

"I could help Sally know about things she didn't know about to keep her safe."

"How did you do that?"

"Listening to everyone. Figuring things out."

"Is Sally listening?"

"She was. Not now."

"Why not?"

"I don't think she's ready to know so much. I know stuff she might not want to hear. Stuff she doesn't know yet. I might need help with that...I think it's okay for her to know, but other states are afraid for her to know."

"I certainly appreciate you letting me know. Before we talk more about that, is there a state that might be able to join us—a state that could help Sally know about stuff?"

"Maybe. I mean, I think so."

"We have time—I can wait."

"Okay."

"Hi."

Another voice.

"Hi. Thank you for speaking up. Can you tell me who you are?"

"Sarah."

"Hi Sarah. Thank you for coming to help. Do you know how old you were when you were born?"

"Of course I know. I'm not stupid. I was ten. My job was to hate them all."

"Oh, I know you're not stupid—sorry if that's what it felt like."

"Thanks."

"Do you mean you hated Sally's family?"

"Yes. I hate them all."

"How was that helpful?"

"Because Sally couldn't hate them. She needed them. I didn't. She would get in trouble."

"Oh, I see—that makes a lot of sense. You could hold the hate because you didn't need them? Do you know why you hated them?"

"Are you kidding?"

"No—I'm sorry, again, if it feels like that. I'm working on trying to understand what happened and how you helped."

"I hated them because they were all horrible. Mean. Cruel. They did awful things. I think that's why Sally feels dizzy and like she might be in trouble."

"Because she might be in trouble for knowing things?"

"Yes. It was always safer for her not to know things. It's going to be hard for her to know these things. But can I tell you something I think only I think?"

"Yes—please tell me."

"I think it's time for Sally to know things."

"And it would be hard for her because of how much trouble that would get her into?"

"Yes."

"Can you tell me about the things?"

"Lots of things. Painful things. How they hated her. Especially him. It was really bad for her. The thing that is going to be really painful for her, Dr. Siegel, are the—and I'm going to kind of whisper this because I don't want her to hear it so loud—it'll be scary for her—the sexual things."

"Who is 'him'?"

"You know."

"I'm not sure I do."

"Can I whisper it to you?"

"Yes."

"The father."

"And Sally doesn't know about the father or about the sexual things?"

"She's beginning to know."

"She's listening?"

"Kind of. It's hard for her. I think you better talk to Sally now because I should leave."

"All right, Sarah. Before you go, do you know why her father hated her?"

"No. I don't think she's ready for that."

"Thank you so much for helping. Can I ask one more thing before you go?"

"Sure."

"Can you work with Allison to make sure no harm comes to Sally or any other state?"

"Yes. Allison and I are used to working together."

"I'm so happy to hear that. I look forward to speaking to you again soon, will that be okay with you.?"

"Yes. Okay."

"Thank you and thank Allison."

"Okay. Bye."

Some silence and then Dr. Siegel said,

"Whenever you're ready to come back, Sally, we can talk about what just happened."

It took me a little time to get back in the room. Like I was swimming to the surface. Holding my breath for a long time. Eyes closed. Swimming in the dark. Maneuvering to stay out of the grip of the riptide. I was feeling the terror. Warning, warning. And something I hadn't felt before. Or at least not in a long time. It took me a while to understand what it was. An awful feeling. It wasn't bad about them. It was something bad about me.

"Hi. It's me. Sally. I feel awful, Dr. Siegel."

"I know. Did you hear that?"

"Enough to know that something bad is going to happen. It feels like a battle inside to decide what I can and can't know. Like I'm not in charge. Like I don't get to know what I need to know."

"I understand. We will take it slow, Sally. Did you hear me talking to Sarah?"

My head was spinning.

"Yes. And Allison. That was weird."

"Did you hear them promise no harm?"

"I know. That's good." I was feeling so exhausted.

"You know how we have talked about updating your files?"

"Yes."

"Do you think it would help to consider that the feeling that something bad is going to happen is implicit? And to consider that, even when the awareness of something bad happening is strong, it may be an implicit memory, and allow it to enter and stay in awareness?"

Dr. Siegel explained the idea of widening my window of tolerance. "We all have a window of tolerance for certain things. When we stay stuck within the window, or when the window's too narrow, it can create rigidity. And then if we get overwhelmed by a feeling, it can catapult us out of our window so that we land in chaos. To lessen that, we want to practice sitting with the uncomfortable feelings for even just a short time, which will help to expand our window of tolerance for that particular feeling."

Chaos and rigidity. It did seem to describe what I'd so often felt in our sessions.

"Then when I get wind of the feeling of the bad thing happening, if I can tolerate it for a little bit instead of shutting it down or disappearing, I can widen my window of tolerance for it?"

"That's the idea."

"That makes sense. I can try it."

"Wonderful."

We both just sat there for some time. I knew it was getting close to the end of our session. He always gave me plenty of time to ground myself before having to drive home.

"If it's helpful for you, go ahead and start opening your eyes now—take some breaths...it's time to get ready to wrap up for today."

It was hard to look at him. It was hard for me to have him see me. I just wanted to hide—to keep my eyes closed, and then, when I opened them, to keep the pillow in front of my face. I wanted to protect him from seeing me. Then I thought about my window of tolerance.

"It's hard for me to look at you—so I want to try to just sit here for a couple of minutes to widen my window."

"Let me know if I can help."

"What I'm sitting with is that I don't want you to see me."

"Okay. Well, if you can—stay with that for a little bit. Let it come into awareness."

"Okay."

"Would it help you for me to close my eyes?"

I so appreciated that. I knew I needed to work through this. Wanted to work it through.

"No. It's hard. But thank you."

"What makes it hard?"

"Knowing what's to come. I can't even say it. But I'm sitting with it."

"Say what?"

"What we're going to find out. What you're going to know about me. I can't say it."

"Can you write it to me?"

"Maybe. If I can't say it, but can write it, is that kind of like sitting with it and widening the window?"

"Yes—I think it is."

He handed me a piece of paper and his pen. It took a little while and then I wrote it down. Just one word. A word I couldn't say out loud. I was filled with the bad feeling. I handed it to him. I still couldn't look at him.

"I just can't say it, Dr. Siegel."

"It's okay. You don't have to say it. Can I look at what you wrote?"

"Yes."

He looked at it. Looked at me—I glanced up at him—my quiet tears flowing. Kind, compassionate face. He handed me some more Kleenex.

I was able to pull it together enough to get ready to leave. I put my sunglasses on and was walking toward the office door.

"Are you able to tell me what makes it so hard to say this word to me?"

"I'm not just afraid, Dr. Siegel. There's something else I'm feeling. It's a terrible feeling. I hate it. I'm afraid of what it means about me. I'm afraid for you to know this about me."

I wanted to hide and scream.

"Can you tell me the feeling?"

I sat back down on the couch.

"Feels like I want to crawl inside of myself to hide. That I need to disappear. Like I'm dirty. Contaminated. I hate my body."

"Like you're in danger?"

"No—like I just don't want anyone to see me. Or to know me. Especially you. I don't want you to see me. I don't want you to know this about me."

"Because I've read the word, Sally?"

"Because I can't stand that word. I hate it."

There was a pause. I was trying to gather myself to go. He could sense that there was more, and he asked me to let him know what I was thinking.

"It feels catastrophic. Like the word is a bad word about me."

In the most direct but gentle, "the truth is your friend" way, he answered me:

"It *was* catastrophic, Sally—it's no longer catastrophic. Implicit memory, remember, can come in the form of pure emotion—pure fear, terror, rage, shame."

Shame.

"Is this feeling shame, Dr. Siegel?" I'd never thought about shame.

"I think it might be," he told me.

"Why does it feel so bad?"

"Shame is the feeling not that something is bad, but that *you* are bad. It's a destructive feeling, one that takes hold when parents who are supposed to take care of you don't. When they're the source of shameful acts. I think a state may have been created to make you believe something was wrong with you so that you could feel safe with your parents."

"It was like there was something bad about me, not them?"

"Exactly."

"So catastrophic," I said. That was the word that kept coming to mind.

"It was so catastrophic, Sally, that your brilliant child's mind fragmented and formed memory barriers between states—and that's what saved you."

"So, this feeling of shame is a state, or like a state, that kind of took all the blame for the word I can't say happening? Like it was my fault, not the parents'?"

"I believe so. And—it will feel catastrophic, Sally, as you and I explore the different states—going toward the fear, terror, shame, sadness, grief. But widening your window—that's what will allow you to integrate what happened, dissolving the memory barriers, making it possible for you to know what happened and that it was catastrophic without feeling it any longer."

"I'll just know it?"

"Yes."

"And not feel it. Not get stuck in chaos or rigidity?"

"That's right."

"So, like—I'll remember that I felt shame or terror as a kid, but not feel it anymore?"

"Exactly."

More silence. Both of us taking in this very intense and informative session.

"Dr. Siegel"—I had to ask—"what if I'm not strong enough to know it all? What if I can't survive remembering and knowing any of it?"

There was a rather long silence in the room, but I could feel his absolute presence resonating there with me. He put his notebook down, and with it the piece of paper on which I'd written the word I couldn't say. He was careful to place it face down so I wouldn't see it.

He kept his eyes on me with so much compassion I could feel it. He knew my pain and despair. He had seen it, but he wasn't absorbing it, and it wasn't hurting him. He was right there alongside me with it, metaphorically holding my hand. When he finally did speak, he said the most profound thing anyone had ever said to me:

"You've survived, Sally. You survived."

I hadn't thought of it like that. It was an incredible thing to hear. I was scared, but I would be okay. I had survived it already.

I've survived.

Sex. That was the word I couldn't say. The word I wrote.

I couldn't say it, but I was feeling it all over. Like my body was smoldering, my genitals ablaze. It was excruciating. I think maybe that is the feeling that would so often send me to dive in the ocean within. Go as deep as possible. Cool the body off. It was like if I didn't, the feelings were not just going to drive me crazy...they were going to burn me alive. As if my body wasn't just filled with poison— my body *was* poison. Poisonous. Flammable. Explosive. Warning! Warning! I wanted to hide, but the hiding places were disappearing. I wanted to disappear—but I didn't. I couldn't. I could stay there and know even what I didn't want to know, because I'd survived it. I could be there with it.

Widening the window.

His soothing words were playing on a loop in my mind, like a piece of favorite music. *You're not crazy Sally...You survived...Your brilliant child mind saved you...MPD saved you...We will go slow...I will be with you every step of the way...You will be safe in this office...You are far from crazy.*

Breakthrough.

PART 2

LEAVING DR. SIEGEL'S OFFICE THAT FRIDAY, going to get Sam from preschool, I was working hard to stay grounded—not just for myself but for Sam and Paul. After such an intense week in therapy, I was exhausted and looking forward to the weekend. We didn't have any plans—just us at home. Paul would be going on location soon for his next project—and while Sam and I would certainly visit him, it was the first time he'd be away since we brought Sam home from Romania, and so it was the first time I wouldn't be joining him for the entire run of the film.

I loved being at Sam's school. It sat on a hilltop not far from our home. The playground overlooked the ocean. I loved seeing all the children playing—and of course Sam. Jungle gym. Playhouse. Swings. Treehouse. All the signs of happy, thriving, cared-for, loved children. I couldn't help but think about the contrasts between this, and where I came from—and where Sam had started his life. In essence, I believe that's what had sent me to Dr. Siegel. Going to Romania, to an orphanage full of babies with no one to care for them. It had stirred something in me that needed to be addressed, and thanks to the work I was doing with Dr. Siegel, I was doing what was necessary. My inspiration was to be a good mom. That was the most important and meaningful thing. But I was doing something important for myself, too—and my child self.

After I'd picked Sam up, we stopped at McDonald's for a snack, as usual on our Fridays. Then we headed home, our dogs Bix and Cleo greeted us, and Sam sat down for his Happy Meal. He told me all about his day. He loved school, was learning a lot, becoming more social and athletic. He was a happy child. I was a happy mom. When he finished his snack, we went out the back door to let the dogs play on the beach for a while.

It was something we'd done the first day we brought Sam home from Romania. We'd flown directly from Bucharest via Frankfurt to LAX and home to Malibu, where Paul took Sam and the dogs right out the back gate to the beach. Lots of kids as young as Sam was then—sixteen months—are afraid, hearing the loud roar of the ocean. But Sam, with his blonde ringlets and blue eyes, sat down on the sand with his dad, looked all around him, scooped up a handful of sand, and put it directly in his mouth.

That was the most wonderful day.

We headed back inside—me to the kitchen to start prepping for dinner, Sam watching *Sesame Street*. A little later, when Paul got home from work, I could see he looked tired.

"Tough day at the office?" I asked him.

"A little—you know, movie stuff. How about you? Looks like you may have had a tough day at the office too?"

I loved this about him. Paul was the most optimistic person I'd ever known. Nothing seemed insurmountable to him, and he was always able to bring some humor to the most difficult situations. For Paul, life was an adventure.

"Yes..." I said, "...an especially intense day today."

"Anything you want to talk about? That I might help with?'

Kind of nodding toward Sam in the corner watching his show, I quietly said, "Yes—let's talk later—after Sam goes to bed."

He came over to me, gave me a little hug and kiss and said, "Okay. Sounds good, honey. I'm just going to go up and shower—unwind a little before dinner."

I hugged him back. I knew he had a lot on his mind—this current project was starting up soon and he had a lot to get done before the production went on location. One of the many things I so admired about Paul was not just how good he was at his job, but how much he loved it. I was sorry Sam and I wouldn't be able to be with him the entire time, but knew he understood, and knew where he thrived most was on a movie set.

We ate dinner, spent some family time together, and then I went upstairs with Sam to his room for bedtime. A bit later, Paul joined us as we read stories. Bedtime wasn't so easy for Sam then. He was afraid for us to leave him alone—which made sense, considering how alone he'd been the first sixteen months of his life—so we'd stay with him until he fell asleep. Eventually, he did. So peaceful.

The day was winding down for us, too. I was exhausted from therapy—it'd been a really emotional session. The thing about the word I couldn't say was hovering over me. I hadn't had trouble with that word before I started therapy. Just thinking about it made me feel a little paralyzed.

"Will it help to tell me about your day, Sal?"

Paul and I had talked about how for me, therapy was private. Not something to keep from him—not a secret—a process that unfolded in Dr. Siegel's office where I was working on making sense of myself for myself. It felt like until I understood what was happening, how could I share it with anyone else, even Paul? I just didn't have the words yet. I so appreciated him understanding that and never pushing me to talk about things. But I was understanding something better now after this last session —I understood that there were shifts in my own awareness of my different states of mind. I know that Paul had told Dr. Siegel that he hadn't noticed anything like that—my behavior shifting in ways he found out of character—but I had a feeling that soon he might. I wanted to give him a heads up.

"You know, Paul—I'm becoming aware of something I want to tell you about."

He sat down on the sofa next to me in our bedroom.

"You know, when Dr. Siegel first told me about the diagnosis—my diagnosis, of MPD—he described it as my mind fragmenting, when I was a little kid, to keep me from knowing what I couldn't know, because I was just a little kid. And that makes so much sense to me. And it's like, the only thing I ever knew about MPD before was from that Sally Field movie, *Sybil*, and it never felt like I had *that*—like I had outwardly different personalities with different wardrobes and things."

"Of course. I've never noticed anything like that either, Sally."

"For me, what I'm realizing now is there's an internal process—an internal awareness of different states of mind, that are slowly getting comfortable with Dr. Siegel—comfortable enough to let me know about what happened to me as a kid...And now it feels like I'm waking up from a deep sleep and realizing I don't know anything about my history, where I come from and what happened to me. I feel dazed and lost much of the time."

What's going on with me?

Paul just got closer and hugged me.

"It's really hard for you, Sally, I know."

"Thank you."

"How can I help—especially with me being gone soon?"

"I love you, Paul. I think I'll be fine. I just need time and space to figure all of this out. It's scary, but I'm not really scared to know more even as it does get scarier. I know that's weird to say. But it's how I feel."

"I think I understand, Sally. I think you're incredibly brave. And I think Dr. Siegel is exactly the right doctor to help you. It seems he helps you feel safe."

We spent more time talking—a little more about me; some about the movie, the location he'd be going to, and all that it would entail for him. Where he'd be living. Us coming to visit. I didn't tell him about the word I couldn't say. As so often happened with what went on in therapy, I simply didn't have the words. I couldn't even say the word or all that I'd felt out loud to Dr. Siegel in the session. It was hard enough to think it. To know it. To remember it. It made me glad I'd been able to write it for him.

I climbed into bed first and then Paul a little later. We were cuddling, as we always did. And then Paul made a move to be sexual. We hadn't had sex in a couple of weeks, but it was always fine. Now something happened to me that had never happened before with Paul—I froze. I mean, I couldn't move. He was startled for sure. Asked me what was wrong, and the quiet tears began to flow. I just couldn't. I couldn't. *I'm sorry, Paul, I just can't. Please don't be mad. Please don't be hurt. I'm sorry. I love you. I can't. I don't know why.* I just felt blank. Lost. I knew I was there, but I felt I was not. I felt myself curl into the fetal position. As I drifted off, I could hear Paul saying, "It's okay, Sally...Are you okay?...Should I call Dr. Siegel?...Do you see him on Monday?..." But I fell asleep before I could answer that yes, yes, I do see him on Monday.

I don't think he understood what had happened, even after the conversation we'd had. How could he? I didn't really either. So confusing. It must've been strange for him, or worse. I was trying my best to be normal, even with these things going on with me in therapy that I had no ability to talk about, that I could barely make sense of yet—but things weren't normal for me. Paul was never angry, unkind, or intrusive; he trusted me to do what was needed and he respected my need to work this out on my own time. I don't think he felt helpless. But I do believe he knew he couldn't help except just to be there. And I was in no shape to help him understand—I was grateful he was seeing his own therapist. It was simply a time in which we both had to just deal with what came as best we could.

Next thing I knew, Paul was hovering over me in bed, gently shaking me and saying, softly enough not to wake Sam in his room across the hall, but forcefully enough to get me to open my eyes:

"Sally, sweetheart, wake up...Hey, you're having a bad dream. Come on. It's okay. Are you okay? Wake up."

I opened my eyes and was filled with terror and confusion. Paul was right there.

Thank you, Paul, thank you for always being right there.

"I'm okay, I'm okay. Thanks. It's okay. I'm sorry."

"You sure?"

"Yes, Paul—you go back to sleep. I'm going to go downstairs to try and settle a little, write in my journal. Maybe get back to sleep...you go back to sleep. It's okay—just another bad dream. And yes...I do see Dr. Siegel Monday...if I need I'll call him—but I'm okay..."

I knew what was ahead of me, and it didn't include sleep. Since my diagnosis, and the intensity of therapy, especially since visiting my parents, I'd been having regular nightmares, often accompanied with flashbacks. Nearly impossible to get back to sleep. Terrified. Dr. Siegel had suggested that it might be helpful to write down the nightmares and flashbacks as soon as I woke up from them, so we could talk about them in session. So, grabbing my journal, I headed downstairs.

It was in the middle of the night and both the insomnia and the terror were in full force. I was writing in my journal. Trying some of the other tools Dr. Siegel had taught me about. Breath. Hand on heart. Widening the window...

But the flashbacks kept intruding...

Emotions racing through my body and mind.

I hate my body. I hate my body. I hate my body. Did I just feel that, or did a state write it in the Bulletin Board section of my journal? *I don't want to feel. I don't want to feel. I don't want to feel. Please stop. Please stop. Stop. Stop. Stop. I can't stop the feeling...it won't stop. The feeling down there. The word I can't say. Can't say. Can't say. Please stop. Being curious isn't helping. I don't want to know. Don't want to know. Don't know. Won't know. Can't know. The noise. The noise. The noise. I have to stop it. Stop it. Oh...relief...thank you...thank you...no more feeling...okay... better...blank...thank you...thank you...sleep now...*

I was so overwhelmingly aware of my vagina that I thought it would drive me insane.

What the fuck is that feeling?

It was horrible. Haunting. Shame-filled. Painful. It disgusted me. I didn't want anyone to see me. *Please help me. I'm going to hide so deep that you will have to really work hard to find me. Please help me. Please find me. Make it stop. Make it stop. Make it stop. The word I can't say. Can't say. Can't say.* And the noise. So much noise.

It wouldn't go away.

I AWOKE EARLY IN THE MORNING, hoping it was Saturday but realizing it was Sunday and that our weekend was ending, I heard Paul, Sam, and the dogs on the beach. I rarely went in the water much before August, because it was just too cold even with a wetsuit. But this spring morning I couldn't wait to jump into the cold water...I felt my body longing to feel the cold water. I threw my swimsuit on and ran out to the beach and joined Paul who was already in the water. Waving to Sam playing on the deck, I think I startled Paul...

"You okay?"

"I think so. The water feels so good." It felt kind of free. Almost like I could breathe under water. How wonderful that must be.

"You never go in this early."

"Not never—just not lately. It feels good."

He was noticing some of what I was experiencing in my internal world. The shifts. I was so glad I'd been able to tell him a little about it. I think it helped us both.

Later that night Paul and I fell asleep together. Spooning. I told him I was sorry about the other night. He told me he understood.

"Do you think it's something you should bring up with Dr. Siegel?"

"Yes—I think so. I will."

But I knew it would be hard to talk about it with him. I was pretty sure I'd written about it in my journal.

I welcomed the closeness with Paul tonight. It felt good. Normal. Comforting. And there were no nightmares that night. But the dreadful insomnia did arrive, right on schedule. And the flashbacks. The pain-filled, noisy flashbacks. They always hurt my ears.

I DROPPED SAM OFF AT PRESCHOOL and drove down the Coast Highway to Dr. Siegel's office in Brentwood. The office was inviting and comfortable—even the waiting room. I always felt a little nervous before going in, not knowing what was going to come up. But today I was excited to share with him the feeling of swimming, and what it had brought up for me.

"It was exhilarating, Dr. Siegel. I felt like I was a happy little girl. I'm remembering one of the things that made me happy as a kid was to be at the pool we belonged to, in the summer in Chapel Hill. Not the beach so much, because I almost drowned once and couldn't go in alone. But I could spend the whole day at the pool. There was a lifeguard, lots of people, friends. I don't remember my family being around there. I would play mermaid or dolphin. I'm so happy to remember it. I just loved it."

A happy memory. It was nice to have had one of those come up—that didn't happen very often.

Then I told him about the nightmares and flashbacks—the insomnia. I told him that on Friday night after our word-I-can't-say session I hadn't slept well at all and had spent much of my night alone downstairs writing in my journal.

"Do you have it with you?"

"The Bulletin Board?—yes."

"Would it be helpful to take a look?"

I got it out of my bag—opened it up and...well, my happy mood quickly shifted. He could see the shift.

"What's going on?"

Just looking at the pages of handwriting that weren't mine. It wasn't the first time I'd seen it like that, but it was still a jolt, especially in Dr. Siegel's office. As I read through the few pages I'd written since the last time I'd really checked it, there was a lot I hadn't seen before.

It felt disorienting. A wave of confusion came over me. "I need to lie down."

I took my shoes off, grabbed the blanket and pillow and lay down. I closed my eyes and covered my face with the pillow.

There was a very long silence. A long silence. Finally, he spoke:

"Sally, I can't help but notice that there is blood on the feet of your socks."

Shit.

I'm not sure how much time passed before I was able to speak. I was a little frozen...then felt another shift suddenly. Outside in. It was as if the electricity in the room, and in *me*, went out. Heavy eyes. Everything went dark. I was blank.

"I don't think I can talk about this."

"I understand it's hard to talk about, but we need to talk about it."

"Why?"

Again, a long pause.

"It's my job to keep you safe—to do that, I'd like to know about the blood on your socks. Where'd it come from? Do you know?"

"Sort of."

I opened my eyes and could see he wasn't angry or upset, just concerned.

"Sally, I'm hoping you can stay so we can talk about this. If you need to hide, that's okay, but I'd like someone to come let me know about the blood."

I wasn't sure what to do. I was feeling blank and had no real awareness of ...well, of anything.

"When you took your shoes off to lie down, did you know the blood was there?"

"I forgot. I'm really confused."

"Tell me more about being confused?"

I was completely dizzy inside. My thoughts swirling so fast I couldn't follow them. I was upset and didn't know what was happening. I *wanted* to know. I wanted things to make sense. But it didn't seem like I had the ability to know or understand anything. I just wanted to disappear.

Slowly, gradually, words came. "I think something happened over the weekend."

"Can you tell me?"

"I don't want to."

"I know, I know. But we need to. Can you ask for help?"

After a little while...

"Jennifer wants to come help."

"Help or take over?"

"Take over and I can hear."

We agreed that if it was too upsetting I could stop listening. But Dr. Siegel was really hoping I could remain present.

"Hi."

"Jennifer?"

"Yes."

"Thanks for coming to help. How are you?"

"Okay."

"Do you know what happened over the weekend?"

"I do."

"Can you share it with me?"

Yes, she could. Jennifer explained that Paul wanted to have sex.

"It wasn't that Sally didn't want to have sex. She just couldn't."

"Why not?"

Jennifer explained that there was real upset going on internally. There were states that didn't know about each other. States that had been mostly isolated. Alone. Solo. States that had very different experiences with and histories of sex, different feelings about sex, different roles and jobs around sex. Some information was seeping through to these states, and over the weekend, when Paul was in a sexual mood... Sally froze.

"She froze?"

"Yes. She couldn't move. Then she started crying. And she freaked out a little and was kind of asking him not to be mad at her. Not to hate her. I understood it, but I don't think he did."

"What did he do?"

"He fell asleep. And then later, when Sally was screaming from the nightmare, he helped her, and she went downstairs. The insomnia is bad."

"Thanks, Jennifer—I so appreciate your help."

Dr. Siegel was curious about the extent of Jennifer's knowledge about what was going on. She let him know she knew everything. And she could know everything because she never feels anything. She could know because she doesn't feel.

"You don't feel physical things, or emotional things?"

"I don't feel anything. Ever," she said. "But I know everything."

He complimented her on how useful that must've been growing up in that family. How genius to find a way to know everything without having to feel any of it.

Survival.

"Yes."

"Are you able to tell me about the blood on Sally's socks?"

"It's tricky."

"I'd appreciate your letting me know what you can."

Jennifer explained how it worked. Sally could be sexual. She sometimes liked it, and sometimes it was hard for her, but she could. As for the other states, there were lots of states that only deal with sex. There were states that love sex. States that didn't like it. States that hated it. States that were terrified by it. None of them knew about each other, but because of all the work Sally had been doing with Dr. Siegel and all the things she was becoming aware of...about her parents being so abusive...the sex states were getting confused about who should show up. "There's a bunch of them."

"A bunch of states that show up for sex?"

"Yes. Sally got confused about how to feel about having sex with Paul and a bunch of them came at the same time and it freaked her out and she shut down. Froze."

Flashbacks.

Implicit memory.

Memory barriers.

Chaos and rigidity.

Jennifer went on to explain that when Sally was a kid—when things happened so fast and she didn't know who she was going to face, what they were going to do, how they were going to be, and what state she needed—the Just Blank state would step in until whatever state could help would show up.

"The Just Blank state?"

"Yes. The Just Blank state could stand in because it didn't feel anything or know anything. It was numb."

"How's that different from you?"

"The Just Blank state could be numb because it didn't know anything about what was happening. I know but I don't care, so even though I'm not numb I can't be hurt. The blank state doesn't have feeling in a different way...kind of like it's dead."

"Or frozen?"

"Yes."

"You can be indifferent?"

"I think so."

"Okay."

"And when no state could get there to help, the Just Blank state would be there and be numb. And because Sally hates being numb— she cuts herself. When she cuts herself, she feels something. And it kind of feels good. But she never knows why. And she kind of hates herself after."

It's so fucked up.

"Thank you again, Jennifer, for being so helpful. Can you help Sally not cut?"

"I can try. Maybe Allison could help too."

"That would be great. I'd like to ask Sally to come back now."

"Before she does, Dr. Siegel, can I tell you one more thing?"

"Yes, certainly."

"I think I should whisper it."

"All right."

"Dr. Siegel...some of the states that deal only with sex...some of them are really little. Not everyone knows about them."

"Does Sally know about them?"

"She's starting to. She knows there's lots of confusion and sadness and pain and terror about sex. She's having flashbacks of stuff."

"Thanks for letting me know."

"Can I tell you one more thing?"

"Please do."

"A bunch of us think it's time for Sally to know more."

"What makes you believe she's ready?"

"Before more stuff starts to leak out. If she could find out with you, we think that would be better than it just exploding out."

"I thank you for letting me know."

THERAPY WITH DR. SIEGEL WAS PAINFUL, exhilarating, and illuminating. This second year as his patient was about getting to know my states.

I was grateful to have Dr. Siegel, and the many tools he'd taught me—especially now, with the Bulletin Board. It was a gathering place where all the states could meet to communicate with each other, me, and Dr. Siegel. At first it'd been jolting to read things that I didn't recall writing, and not in my handwriting. The states would express all kinds of things—emotions, therapy, internal frustrations, information they wanted to be brought to Dr. Siegel's attention. I got used to it, though, and began to find it so useful that I journaled daily, to keep connecting with the many states that had been born out of my mind's ability to adapt to the abuse of my childhood.

I came to know many of these states quite well. Some made themselves known to me more readily than others; some emerged only painstakingly slowly. It was never easy. Always emotionally painful, and often excruciatingly so. The suffering they reflected sometimes felt too much for me to know or bear—which of course is why they'd come into existence in the first place. Sometimes, their suffering was more from *perceived* danger, and it would take time for me to discern the difference between real, present danger and what had come before—implicit memory. But eventually I would learn when the states had come into existence, what their purpose had been, how they'd helped me survive, and how they at times worked together, and other times worked at cross-purposes. Some hated others. Some were purely purpose-driven; others held emotions in their purest form. Some states had been born of both physical and emotional pain, some out of secrecy, some out of hope, some out of fear, and some out of just a primal drive to survive, to stay alive. There were dreamer states dreaming of a wonderful life ahead. Some states were scared; some scary. Some couldn't speak yet; some only needed sleep. Over time I came to recognize them, and, ultimately, to be grateful to them all.

One of the other things I was most grateful for was Dr. Siegel's telling me that I could call him whenever I needed to.

Sometimes I would need to. He always called me back as quickly as he could. Sometimes I would call just to hear his voice on his answering machine. That could be enough. Sometimes I would leave a message and say I didn't need him to call me back—just connecting this way was enough. After especially difficult sessions, he would ask me to leave a message for him to let him know how I was doing. It always helped.

Outside of therapy I was reading everything I could about MPD, memory, attachment, trauma, PTSD, early childhood abuse, and incest. There. I said it. Another word that for so long I couldn't say. Not to Dr. Siegel, not to myself....I could barely hear it. Hard to accept it happened to me. With Dr. Siegel's help I was learning and understanding its impact on me.

Of course, it's easy to say all this now, in narration. It took a long time to work through all of this in reality.

"The most important thing, Sally, is your safety," Dr. Siegel would often remind me.

That was always the highest priority. The deeper therapy went, the more awareness there was within, and though there were states that were created very much for my safety, there were other parts that were in the dark, not understanding what was going on, not willing to meet Dr. Siegel, creating a great deal of internal chaos and rigidity. There were also states that I was too afraid of to know about yet. That often led to therapeutic stalemates where I felt lost, stuck, hopeless, and afraid.

"We will go as slow as you need to," Dr. Siegel always told me during those impasses.

So far, there had never been any suicidal activity. But the cutting that had started didn't stop. It progressed from the toes to the arms—mostly the right arm. And it was a concern.

Over several sessions, Dr. Siegel noticed, too, that I kept rubbing my right ear. When he asked me about it, I got very quiet and withdrew, much as I'd done when he noticed the blood on my socks. I'd let him know in earlier sessions that the flashbacks I was having at home at night were deeply troubling, and a main feature of those flashbacks was a noise I found intolerable. The noise in the flashbacks and this habit of rubbing my ear: they clearly seemed connected in some way. Dr. Siegel invited any state that might have some information to come forward, but none did—not even Jennifer, Allison, or Sarah. Jennifer said she knew, but didn't want to talk about it. Then, one session, when he asked the question again, a state did appear.

"I can help."

"Thank you. Do you have a name?"

"Not really. Just the state that hates the body.'

"I'm glad to meet you. Can you tell me about hating the body, and what your purpose is?"

"I hate the body. It deserves to be hated. It causes so much pain. I hate it. How can a body be good?"

"Do you know about the noise in flashbacks that Sally's hearing?"

"It's the noise I hate."

"What's the noise?"

"When they're doing things to her."

"What kind of things?"

"The word-she-can't-say things. I can say it, but she hates it."

"So, sexual things?"

Eventually, the state that hates the body was able to tell Dr. Siegel about the flashbacks. The noise was the noise of a little girl having sexual things done to her. "Not the sounds she was making. The sounds they made doing things to her."

"Who is 'she'?"

"Sally."

"Who is 'they'?"

"I can't talk about that."

The telling of the whole story was excruciating. It took many long sessions. It would take many hours and days of therapy for the memory to unfold and be told and known. I couldn't open my eyes. The words were difficult to speak and sometimes to understand. It was torture. Remembering the feelings and sounds of being sexually molested and raped by my father. I was terrified. All the time. No part of my body was safe. My vagina. My mouth. My anus. My ears. The sessions were crushing.

The state that hates the body once told Dr. Siegel, "When the noise gets too hard for Sally, I try to kill the noise."

"The noise in the ear?"

"Yes."

"How do you do that?"

"With a stick."

"What kind of stick?"

"Usually a pencil."

"How does that help?"

"When I stab the ear with the stick, it makes it hurt, which makes the noise go away."

"So, the pain's better than the noise?"

"Uh-huh."

More and more of the details of the abuse surfaced. What Dr. Siegel began to learn was it was the cutting of the toes and the arm and the stabbing of the ear that stopped the pain. It was superficial—only someone seeing me as closely as Dr. Siegel had in that one session when he'd seen my socks would've been able to know I was doing it—but helped to stop the pain.

"I thought the ears were about the noise?" Dr. Siegel asked the state that hated the body.

"The noise is the pain," the state said. "The stick-pain kills the noise pain."

Dr. Siegel asked some more about the cutting and stressed the need for the states to come together to stop all body-harming strategies. No more sticks in the ear. No more cutting. He was curious if there was a state that could help the state that hates the body find a less harmful and dangerous way to ease the pain. The state that hates the body checked inside. After a few minutes, a new state came up:

"Hi. You're Dr. Siegel, right?"

"Yes. Who are you?"

"Nobody."

"Nobody?"

"Yes."

"Really, you're Nobody?"

"Yes."

"Can you tell me how you help?"

"Because I'm Nobody."

"I'm not sure I understand—can you explain more, please?"

"It wasn't safe to have a body in that family, so I'm no body."

"Oh—you're not 'Nobody'—you have *no body*!"

"Yes, I have no body. I'm No-Body."

"I'm sorry I misunderstood."

"It's okay."

No-Body provided relief. When things got so bad and painful for me, No-Body could take over and never experience any pain because it had no body. No vagina. No anus. No mouth. No ear.

As we worked on the pain of the body, more and more states were surfacing—the states that knew, the states that didn't know, states that felt, states that didn't feel. I was getting to know them and to understand how they formed a system to keep me as safe and sane as possible. Often, before a new state appeared, I would be terrified to let it come up, to meet it, or let it meet Dr. Siegel. But he worked with each state and was gradually able to understand why and when they were born. They all had a real purpose. All in service of survival. I was understanding and appreciating that more and more.

Still, some states were particularly terrifying for me.

"I can't let those states come out."

"Can you let me know why?"

"They're so angry." I could feel the intensity of the emotion. It felt enormous and destructive.

"Do you know who or what they're angry about?"

The fear was paralyzing.

"I just know if they come, something bad will happen."

"What bad thing will happen?"

"I'm afraid they'll hurt you."

"What if I let all angry states know that they are welcome to come here, but there is to be no damage to my body or your body or to anything in the room?"

"Do you think that'll work?"

"I think it will. They can punch pillows. They can yell. They can say whatever they want. Just no physical damage to bodies or furniture."

Eventually, with his invitation and his assurance that he believed it would be safe, I was able to let the angry states come to meet him.

What was revealed was the depth of their anger over how much they had endured.

"I hate them."

"Who?"

"The parents. I hate them."

"I understand that. Can you tell me a little more about hating them?" Dr. Siegel asked.

"They do mean things. They hurt us. They hate us. They hate Sally."

"Can you tell me how they hurt you?"

"With their hands. And other things. I don't like to talk about it. Please don't make me talk about it."

"I won't make you. Maybe sometime later you can let me know?"

"Maybe."

"Can Sally come join us to hear about your anger?"

"I'm here."

"How are you feeling about this anger, Sally?"

"I don't know. I don't know what I'm feeling or what to feel. Confused. I feel confused." They weren't what I was expecting. I thought they wouldn't be just angry, but violent. The internal sense I would get felt dangerous, even violent.

"Does it feel dangerous now?"

"Not really—which is not what I was expecting. Why do you think I've been so afraid of the anger, Dr. Siegel?"

"Why do you think?"

"I just don't know."

"Well, it might be that you've mistaken rage, which is what your father had, with anger. Anger, Sally, is a healthy emotion that deserves to be expressed. It's not dangerous at all. Rage is different from anger."

"Right."

"Sally, what would happen when you got angry when you were little?"

"I could never be angry."

"Why not?"

A deep sadness came over me when Dr. Siegel asked me that. Despair. I was glad I was lying down because otherwise I surely would've fainted.

"I feel like I might throw up."

Don't throw up. Don't throw up. Don't throw up.

"Right now?"

"Yes."

Don't.

Dr. Siegel brought the trash can over to me.

I just lay there for a while. Sat with the awareness of what would've happened if I got angry when I was a kid. Terrible things. So, I quickly learned not to get angry. Bury it deep. Scream in my head. Cut. Disappear. Be invisible. Numb my body. Grab a stick and poke it in my ear.

I felt dizzy and woozy. I think I may even have been shaking. And I was hearing the voice.

"What voice?"

I could barely say the words.

"I can't..."

"What makes it hard?"

"It feels dangerous."

"To say the words?"

"To hear the words."

I grabbed my right ear.

"Are you hearing them now?"

"Yes."

"Is it dangerous for you to say them?"

"Dangerous for you to hear them."

"I understand words can be scary, but they won't harm me."

"Promise?"

"Promise."

"The angry states say they can say them with me."

"Does that feel okay?"

"Yes. I think they want to scream."

"Screaming is okay."

So, I put the pillow over my face and screamed into it. And screamed. And screamed. And screamed...and then more tears....

The tears were not quiet anymore. They were pouring out. I was sobbing and I was feeling the power of the truth they'd been trying to protect me from for so long. It was the truth, and I needed to know it—to hear it, feel it, and scream it.

The truth is your friend.

"I'm going to vomit up these words. Her words."

"Who?"

"Her name makes me sick."

"The trash can's right there if you need it."

Quite some time went by. I sat up on the couch. I felt sick and I was crying, and I said the words:

"My mother."

Fuck her.

I didn't vomit. But I did scream the words, her words, burning in my ears.

"I'll burn you alive."

"I'll skin you alive."

"I'll bury you alive."

"I'll slit your throat."

"I'll show you what anger feels like."

"I'll give you something that hurts."

"I'll give you something to cry about."

"I'll show you what to do with that stick."

"I'll beat you to death."

"I'll beat you within an inch of your life."

"I'll split you up the middle."

Crying. Sobbing.

Who fucking says that to a little kid?

Flashes of her chasing me with a belt. My whole body was stinging. Shaking.

"I'll blister you."

You fucking monster.

Her room. Green blanket. And that smell that makes me sick.

"I'll blister you so hard you won't be able to sit for a month."

"You better get out of my sight if you want to live."

Swinging the belt at me. Hitting me. All over.

Who fucking does this to anybody, much less a kid?

Chasing me with a wooden yard stick. Hitting me everywhere.

Dragging me to the sink by my hair and jamming a bar of soap down my throat washing my mouth out for what I had said.

What the fuck had I said?

It was the first time I had clear, visual memories of her hurting me.

It was her.

I fucking hate her.

I hadn't thought it was her. For so long, I'd thought it was me. I thought there was something wrong with me.

I fucking hate her.

You don't miss what you never had.

I fucking hate her.

I hope you don't find out it was Mom.

I OPENED MY EYES A LITTLE and looked at Dr. Siegel and he looked disgusted. I was afraid at first he was disgusted with me. But I realized he was disgusted with her. Not me. And not simply disgusted with her. He was angry. Maybe even enraged.

"You know Sally, she could've been—should've been—arrested for her treatment of you."

We talked about it for a long time.

"We've talked about this before, Sally. Sometimes children who grow up with abusive parents will find a way to blame themselves for all the bad things happening. It's a protective measure. A kid can feel safer if the bad things are because of them. If the parents are to blame, well, that makes it hard for a child to survive."

I got up and moved the trash can back to its rightful place.

"I don't need this, but thanks." The feelings of sickness had passed.

"You're welcome. It would've been fine if you had."

"I just needed to get the words out.'

"Yes. What did it feel like to say those words?"

"It feels better now. I understand their anger now."

"Whose anger?"

"The angry states."

I found myself laughing a little.

"What's that?"

"My anger. It's my anger. I know they kept me safe by keeping it inside. Thank you, angry states. Thanks for keeping me safe. Thanks for letting it out."

"Good."

"It's hard to know she did that. I guess I just thought it was what mothers did."

"Have you ever done that to Sam?"

"Oh god no."

"How little do you think you were when this started?"

I had a flash of memory of my mother dragging me to the sink in the kitchen in Washington. It made me flinch.

"I think by around four."

"When you get home, Sally, I want you to really take a close look at Sam—he's about the age you were then—and remind yourself you were that little when she was doing that. You were a child. You were as little as Sam is now."

WHEN I GOT HOME THAT DAY, Sam was with our babysitter. As soon as he saw me he got excited—"Mommy's home!"—and ran to show me a toy he was playing with.

I scooped him up and held him close. Gently. Lovingly. Protectively. Safely.

"I love you, Mommy."

"I love you, Sammy! I missed you this afternoon! I'm so happy I'm home with you now!" He was such a happy kid. I put him down and he went back to playing with his toys.

He was so little. *I'd* been so little. How could anyone hurt a child? Over and over again? They were monsters, my parents.

I fucking hate her.

THE FIRST THING I TOLD DR. SIEGEL at the start of our next session was:

"At first, some of the angry states felt mean and dangerous even. I felt afraid of the things they felt and said—afraid of them—but once they came out, I could see they were just scared or confused little kids and that's why they were so angry. They were so little. I want to let them know how sorry I am they had to go through all that. And I'm sorry I thought they would hurt me. Sorry I thought they'd hurt you."

"Yes, Sally—and you were so little, too. I'm sorry you had to go through that. I wish I could have been there for you then."

Me too.

SOMETIME AFTER THOSE SESSIONS, something happened that let me know that my mother's voice was still somewhere inside of me. It was a weeknight; Paul and I were having a few friends over for dinner. Sam was also having his very first sleepover at our place with his best friend, Molly. The two of them were really bonded. The sleepover was such a milestone event that Molly's mother had made them matching pajamas. Before we sat down for dinner, I went up to Sam's room to get the kids settled for bed. After I said goodnight and turned out the light, Molly started crying and said she needed to go home—she missed her mom. She wasn't ready to sleep away from mom and home. Although I was very sorry to disappoint Sam, I went downstairs and called Molly's parents to let them know Paul would be driving her home.

As Paul was on his way out the door with Molly, Sam said he wanted to go with his dad to Molly's.

I said, "No, it's cold and rainy—you need to stay here."

Paul took Molly and off they went to get the car. But Sam insisted he wanted to go with Daddy.

"No, Sam, it's time for you to go back to bed."

But once I put him in bed, he jumped out, still insisting, "I want to go with Daddy!"

"No! In bed!"

He was jumping out of bed, and I was not-so-gently putting him back. I wasn't hurting Sam, and I certainly didn't want to, but I could have. I was also hearing a loud, angry voice within, saying, *Sam needs to learn when Mommy says no, she means no. Sam needs to learn that no means no.*

And I could hear another somewhat quieter voice whispering, *What are you doing, Sally?*

"Loud and angry" drowned out quiet whispers.

Eventually Sam jumped out of bed, grabbed a large plastic container full of crayons and smashed it in my face. My nose immediately started bleeding. I was crying, Sam was crying, and when Paul got home and came upstairs to see what was going on, he—and our three dinner guests, who'd been downstairs the whole while, unaware—were upset with Sam. Horrified that he'd hit me, that he'd done something violent.

I went to the bathroom across the hall to wash my face, and when I came back to Sam's room, I saw him walking in circles around his little table and chairs, crying, "I love my mommy, I love my mommy, I love my mommy..."

And I didn't know what to do. I realized I had Dr. Siegel in the morning, and something in my head was screaming that I knew what he was going to tell me—that they must've been wrong at UCLA, and there really was something wrong with Sam.

But I could also see that Sam was so upset. So, I picked him up, hugged him and took him to sleep with his dad and me. It was hard for me to fall asleep that night—I just held Sam until he was sound asleep.

I woke up the next morning with a very bruised and messed-up face. When I got to Dr. Siegel's office and he saw me, he asked me what had happened. I told him the whole story. He listened as he always did, and I never detected any alarm in his demeanor. He sat back in his chair, and said,

"You do need to talk to Sam about how hitting is never a good option. But first, Sally, I have to ask you something..."

"What?"

"Why couldn't Sam go with his dad to take Molly home?"

Another stunning moment of awareness for me. Letting Sam go with his dad after I had said no had never once occurred to me.

Reluctantly—sheepishly—I replied, "Because when Mommy says no, no means no."

Oh god. It was hitting me what had happened, that I'd been operating on implicit mental models that were the very opposite of who I wanted to be as a mother.

"Can you see how you kind of backed him into a corner? He's so small—Molly's his best friend—this was his first sleepover ever. Sounds like he was heartbroken."

Yes, yes—of course. Heartbroken. Heartbreaking.

Ugh.

"You know, I had this awareness of a voice saying, *Sam needs to learn that when mommy says no, no means no.* And I had this other awareness: *Why are you doing this?*"

"What voice was saying 'no means no'?"

Deep breaths....

"My mother's."

"No doesn't have to always mean no. It's okay to be flexible as a parent. Sometimes no does mean no—'No, you can't run out into the street.' But Sam was showing you he was really struggling. Even though it was a cold and rainy night, and even though you'd at first said no, it would've been okay to change your mind and bundle him up to go with his dad to take Molly home."

Of course. I felt like a terrible mother for not knowing it and told Dr. Siegel so. He said, "You know Sally, you're only human. We all make mistakes with our kids. Ruptures with our children are inevitable. The important thing is to make the repair. The repair is crucial, and a golden opportunity, really. But being kind to yourself is important too. Learn from this."

We also talked more about the window of tolerance. My window. On the sleepover night, I'd gotten rigidly stuck in my being right, Sam being wrong, and when he "defied" me, I got shot out of my window of tolerance right into chaos. BOOM!

"Wow. Such a lesson. I think what happened last night in Sam's room was my childhood hijacking my brain and attempting to drag Sam and his childhood back into mine."

"What was it like to hear your mom's voice like that?"

"It was scary. And I can only imagine what it was like for Sam to see and hear me that angry and mean. Awful for him."

"I'm sure it was upsetting for him. Making the repair with him will be good for you both. And this will give you a couple of things to practice—not just widening your window of tolerance for flexible parenting but widening it around the fears you have about something being wrong with Sam. Sam is fine. Things will go wrong as you're parenting him, but that doesn't mean there's anything wrong with Sam. Remember—that is what brought you in to see me originally. Nothing was wrong with Sam—it was something that was very wrong in your childhood. Not Sam's. Sam's having a good childhood."

Sam's having a good childhood.

With that, I was out of his office and on my way home to let Sam know that it's never okay to hit people—but that *I* had been wrong not to change my mind about letting him go in the car to take Molly home, once I saw how important it was to him.

"I was wrong to get so angry. I'm sorry, Sammy. So sorry I scared you like that."

"I'm sorry I hurt your nose, Mommy. I love you."

"I love you too."

I love you so much.

WHEN I BEGAN THERAPY, I had no idea what lay ahead of me. Two years in, after one of the toughest but richest, most productive periods of my life, I knew there was still work to be done, but I had a much better idea of what the process involved. We'd come along far enough that Dr. Siegel and I were starting to reflect on the work we'd done and what was ahead.

"I can tell things are changing, Dr. Siegel."

"Tell me about that."

I took a few minutes to gather my thoughts.

"That I feel better. That I'm getting better."

He was curious to know what "better" meant.

"Even though what we're working on is hard, painful—sometimes even shocking—I'm not that shocked by it anymore. I know my childhood was bad, and I really want to know everything so I can free myself from it all. The things that've been so confusing for so long aren't anymore."

"That's great, Sally. It sounds like more than ever, you're able to learn and know what happened to you—and that's what making sense is. Not making sense of your family's actions, but understanding the impact it's had on you."

"And the impact of their actions for me was MPD?"

"Yes."

"Now what?"

"We keep working. The more you know, the more you're able to hold in awareness all that you discover without being thrown into chaos or rigidity...and that is what trauma resolution is."

"To know everything that happened, and it will just be...what happened...not what's happening?"

"Yes."

"No longer intrusive like with dreams and flashbacks?"

"Yes, Sally."

"What about the states?"

"I think you can see already that the internal communication between the states we know about is more open and fluid."

"Yes."

"As the states become more known and connected, the memory barriers your mind created to protect you will dissolve."

"Because I no longer need to be protected from the past because I survived and can know about it?"

"Yes."

"And by resolving my trauma, and the memory barriers dissolve, I don't have MPD any longer?"

"That's right."

"What will that feel like?"

He took a few minutes to answer.

"I think it will feel like you have all the knowledge, tools, and wisdom of the states without the separations."

"But what will it feel like? How will I know it?"

"I think you'll know it, Sally, when it happens. I think you'll have a clarity of mind, deep wisdom about your whole life, and a sense of energy that will be unmistakable."

"And then I'll be recovered from MPD?"

"Yes. Once the trauma is resolved by your making sense of it, and you no longer have memory barriers—yes, we can call that recovery."

Hopeful.

THINGS WERE HAPPENING OUTSIDE OF THERAPY, too, offering me opportunities to work on widening my window of tolerance for difficult situations.

In the fall of 1993, two emergency situations occurred. The first happened while Paul was shooting a film in Russia. I was watching the news from home when I saw a report that riots were breaking out in Moscow, right where Paul was. The Russian White House—a prominent government building—was being burned. And suddenly on the news they had an American, right across from the burning building, giving an off-camera, blow-by-blow eyewitness report of the unfolding unrest. It was Paul! It was alarming to hear his voice so near the danger—but I didn't feel that alarm in an overwhelming, all-encompassing way. It felt like the kind of concern for his safety that anyone in my situation would have. While it would take some hours, eventually he got through to me by phone to say he was safe.

Barely a month later, with Paul still in Moscow, we had one of the worst fires ever to hit Malibu. Malibu had lots of fires, but this was the first time my neighborhood was ordered to evacuate. It was an extreme, urgent situation, and I had only minutes in which to prepare to leave—just enough time to gather Sam, our pets, and our most important documents, which were Sam's Romanian adoption records and his US naturalization papers.

It took us a few hours to get out of Malibu because the roads were jammed and blocked and there was a lot of panic. It was the middle of the day, yet the sky was black with smoke and ash, and you could see flames everywhere—up and down the Coast Highway, and all along the hills and through the canyons. For a brief time, I wasn't sure how we were going to get out, and I remember one moment when I thought we might burn up right there on the road. Frightened as I was, I wasn't hijacked by implicit, past fears. I may have dissociated into the just-blank place a few times, but I did have some awareness that it was happening.

And we didn't burn. We got out safely. And though many of our friends lost their homes, and the fires came so close to our house that for a moment, when watching the news, I thought I might well witness our house go up in flames, it didn't. Nor did I think I would have fallen apart if it did. I had Sam and our beloved dogs, and I knew Paul was safe in Moscow. We rode the time out with friends in Santa Barbara about an hour away, but safe from the fires. Sam and I were happy to get home after a few days.

I was anxious to reach Paul in Moscow—I wasn't sure he knew about the fire; he'd be upset if he did and didn't hear from me. It took hours to get through, and when I did, I reassured him Sam and I and the pets were fine. Again, I don't know how well I'd have handled all this if I hadn't been as far along in therapy as I was.

I'd been able to discern between what was dangerous in the moment and what had been dangerous in the past. I was able to allow my protector mother self to do her job and I didn't collapse like a little child myself in the midst of danger I couldn't control. It was quite a good feeling, even in moments which were quite legitimately terrifying.

I was fully present.

My files were updating.

ONE DAY I SHOWED UP for our appointment and as soon as I entered the office I went straight for the couch, put my bag on the chair next to me, covered myself with the blanket, and closed my eyes. Nearly sixty minutes later, almost as if I'd set an alarm clock, I woke up. We had an hour left.

Dr. Siegel didn't seem alarmed or concerned. When I woke up, he was sitting behind his desk.

He asked me what was going on.

"I just needed to sleep."

"Seems like it."

I had been noticing some internal rumblings and hadn't slept so well the last few nights. Not insomnia—that had subsided. Restless sleep.

"I've been drawing a lot."

As part of my therapy, Dr. Siegel had suggested I use the exercises in a book, *Drawing on the Right Side of the Brain* by Betty Edwards, to stimulate access to my brain's right mode—where autobiographical activity, nonverbal communication, and an integrated map of the whole body are processed. The exercises unleashed a great need and drive to draw and afforded me an artistic skill I had never before known. I had been filling sketchbooks and already had over a dozen. I'd even taken to drawing some of Sam's favorite cartoon characters and teaching him and his friends how to draw them. We were having fun with it.

"Can I show you what I've been drawing?"

"Please do."

I grabbed the sketchbook out of my bag to show him. It was full of pencil and charcoal drawings of little girls. I'd used color pencils on some to highlight their hair and eyes. Sad little girls. Bruised little girls. Little girls with swollen eyes. Girls in tears. Girls in dirty clothes. Disheveled. Sad.

"Tell me about these."

"Just sad and hurt little girls."

"Where do they come from?"

"They kind of draw themselves."

"Why do you draw some of them with a little color?"

"I'm not sure why. I just did. Looking at them now though, even though they look so sad and lost, I think the touch of color conveys their hope."

He pointed out that the color I added was yellow to their hair and blue to their eyes.

"Oh yeah—you're right. Like me."

"Should we see if they want to come to therapy?"

"It doesn't feel like that yet."

"Do you think they're connected to your needing to sleep here?"

"I don't know. Maybe. I think I just needed to sleep."

"That's okay."

"Maybe they needed to sleep too."

Of course, it was about much more than just needing to sleep. I think I needed to sleep in the safety of his office. Maybe it was the little girls needing to sleep safely in his office, too. Maybe. I hadn't been feeling unsafe lately, but I do believe I needed an extra dose of safety that day. And I think I may have had some awareness, even as I was sleeping, that I was safe there—that nothing bad could happen to me in that office.

On my way out, I got a feeling that the little girls were in fact wanting to meet Dr. Siegel. I started thinking there was more to the nap than I entirely understood.

Yet.

AS I WAS ENTERING MY THIRD YEAR of therapy, there were two big shifts. Literally.

The first was just after the new year. We'd had a good holiday and by mid-January were getting back to daily life. Paul was away location-scouting for a new project. Sam was in kindergarten for a longer day now and loving it. I was full-force in therapy, learning more of my truth and ways to be with it. It was hard, it was painful—the need to know it all was my driving force.

In the early hours of January 17, 1994, I was sound asleep in my bed with the dogs. Sam was in his room. Although he would sometimes crawl in with us, he was happier in his own room these days.

The sound came first. Then the shaking. The rumbling. *Earthquake!* I jumped out of bed and ran into Sam's room. I grabbed him in my arms—he was sound asleep, hadn't registered anything—and ran down the stairs while the house was still shaking...I was too. Then it stopped. Everything was completely dark. No electricity, and the sun hadn't come up yet. I realized I was barefoot and had no flashlight...so much for earthquake preparedness. I made my way—Sam still in my arms, barely awake—outside. I could see my neighbors walking with flashlights and started to follow them. We were all headed to the neighbors down the street who we all knew were earthquake prepared. They were ready for us. We all huddled inside their house, waiting for the sun to rise.

When the sun came out, everyone made their way back to their homes to check out the damage. The house we'd gathered in seemed to have none. At all. When I got to our house—same. Not even a fallen plate or a picture frame askew. It was amazing. I got dressed. Sam got dressed. We were just walking around in a bit of a daze. While waiting for sunlight at our neighbors, we'd talked with the kids about the earthquake. How did they feel about it? They were busy figuring out which house to play at after breakfast, excited not to have to go to school! They felt safe and cared for.

As best I can recall, we were without power for a day or two. But some people had battery-operated radios and could hear the news. There was damage in parts of LA—lots. The epicenter was in Northridge, in the Valley; Santa Monica was also hit hard. But Malibu was reporting minimal damage.

I must've missed a week's worth of appointments in that post-earthquake time. I was hoping Dr. Siegel and his office were safe. But the city was kind of shut down. It was hard to get around. Everything was very quiet, and we spent lots of time with our neighbors.

I remember being calm, mostly. Again, I'm not sure how I would have handled this pre-therapy. Especially with Paul gone again. Would I have been hysterical? Checked out? Invisible? Blank? No-Body? I had no way of knowing. I did know, however, that my window of tolerance for unexpected things had definitely widened. As with the fire, I'd been able to focus on our safety. Not worrying about what I didn't know and couldn't control.

Little did I know how soon this widening of my window would come in handy as I faced the next big seismic event in my life.

ONE MORNING, SOON AFTER MY FORTIETH BIRTHDAY and less than a month after what's now known as the Northridge Earthquake, I was driving down the Coast Highway—a notoriously dangerous road—to my appointment when I got this very strange feeling that it would be so easy to drive off the highway.

It came out of nowhere. It wasn't something I'd ever contemplated before. I couldn't find the source of this feeling, either. I couldn't connect it to anything or any state.

"It was a bizarre feeling—an awareness that something could happen," I told Dr. Siegel when I got to his office. "Not something I was thinking before I got in the car this morning. But after the thought showed up, it was hard to get rid of. Does that make sense?"

"Are you having any thoughts or plans to hurt yourself?"

"No, no..."

I could tell this was alarming to Dr. Siegel. I'd never seen him concerned like this.

"Please describe a little more about the feeling you had."

"It felt like...gosh it...it felt..."

I couldn't quite find the right word.

"...it was more of an idea than a thought. But not my idea! It felt random. It felt almost whimsical. Like a whimsy—'Just...you know... hang a right here and off the highway you go.' Almost like for fun. A dare. It was odd."

Saying it out loud now, it felt more real, more threatening than it had when I was driving in. Even dangerous.

"Let's approach this carefully, Sally. Does it feel okay to ask inside what might be going on?"

I closed my eyes to think. I was not looking deep inside this time. It didn't feel like something that called for that. I was feeling frightened, but the fear was different than anything I'd felt in therapy before. Similarly, while I was looking inside, nothing was coming up.

"Tell me what's going on."

"I don't know exactly. It's not like an implicit memory. It feels very present."

Now I was really scaring myself.

"Dr. Siegel..."

"What, Sally?"

Then it hit me.

"I feel like something bad is going to happen. But it's not a feeling from the past. This isn't about something bad from the past. This is something bad that's going to happen in the present. And it's to do with Sam."

Very alarmed now.

Tears.

We were silent for a little while.

"Let's work on figuring this out together, Sally. Can you do that?"

"It feels like I might not ever see Sam again."

"What's going to happen to Sam?"

A very long silence. Tears. Quiet.

"It's not that I'm going to lose Sam, Dr. Siegel. It's that Sam's going to lose me."

He sat there calmly with me.

"Does it feel like you're going to hurt yourself?"

"No. I don't want to die, Dr. Siegel. I've never even thought about that. This is scaring me."

We talked for some time. I think he did come to see that I had no intention of hurting myself. But something was going on. And we needed to figure out what. He didn't want me looking inside for answers either. I think he wanted to keep things calm—not stir anything up.

"We've got some work to do, Sally, to figure this out. Something is going on internally, and I have to keep you safe. I don't think we can work on this with you coming and going up and down that highway while we do it."

"What should I do?"

He took his time, and then finally said, "I want us to do this work in a hospital, where I know you'll be safe."

Hospital? I was shocked. I was alarmed about these feelings and new awareness of danger—and I'd never thought about going away to a hospital, or anywhere. That had never been part of our therapy before.

"When would this happen?"

He said that he'd need some time to figure out the best plan, and it would take some time to make arrangements. But he made a call to somewhere right then. I was just sitting in the chair, in a daze. I could hear him talking about admitting a patient. Non-emergency, but ASAP. Voluntary. Me.

Someone from the hospital would call me later to get my information.

"How long will it be for?"

He took a deep breath and just said, "As long as it takes for us to figure out what's going on with this."

"A few days? A week?"

He didn't answer quickly. I was beginning to get the feeling he was thinking it could be much longer than that.

"I just don't know, Sally. However long it takes to resolve whatever this is. What's concerning you?"

I was still crying.

"I've never left Sam overnight." I wasn't sure it was all about leaving Sam—it just felt very scary to me.

He was incredibly compassionate about it all. We wrapped up the session. But first he wanted assurances from all states that no harm would come to me. Or Sam. That was scary. But with Jennifer and Allison and Sarah's help, he got it.

"See you in the morning," he said. By then we'd know more about how to proceed.

I was still scared as I drove home—but less scared than when I'd driven in. What I kept hearing in my mind was: "The most important thing here, Sally, is your safety. It's my job to keep you safe."

I think he was the only person who had ever said that to me.

IT WAS AWKWARD TELLING PAUL about the hospital. I don't think he really understood—I mean, how could he? How could anyone comprehend what I was experiencing? I believe the abuse I endured and the development of my MPD simply were unfathomable to most. But Paul could see how scared I was, leaving Sam, and he lovingly assured me they'd be fine.

"You've got to do what you need to heal, Sally. If Dr. Siegel and you believe going to the hospital is the right thing, I support that. We'll be fine."

Paul had great faith and trust in Dr. Siegel's treatment of me. Even though we still didn't talk much about therapy at home, it wasn't a taboo subject. By now, it had become routine—a normal part of my life and of our life. And I'd been able to stay grounded through it all, particularly as a mother to Sam. Still, it was also true that between motherhood, MPD, and Paul's being busy working and traveling, the two of us hadn't had a lot of time for any conversations about us lately. But there was no animosity or anger between us, and my sense was we were fine. We'd always been good with each other having different interests and priorities, too. Granted, this was a little different. But I figured that afterward, we'd come together as happily as we'd always done.

Later that day I heard from someone in the admitting office at UCLA Hospital. The woman was asking for my personal information and my insurance information. I don't remember at what point I gathered that she was calling about my being admitted to the psych ward, which was a locked unit.

Locked unit?

"Just what does that mean?"

She let me know it meant I wouldn't be able to come and go as I pleased.

"I don't believe that's what Dr. Siegel was thinking of for me."

She believed it was, and suggested I get in touch with him to clear it up before we went any further.

"I'll talk to him about it tomorrow," I said.

"Let me give you my direct number. Ask him to call me after you decide what to do."

"Thank you."

Locked psych ward? Those words sent shivers throughout my entire body. I knew it couldn't be what Dr. Siegel was thinking.

Still not crazy?

I GAVE HIM THE NUMBER for the woman in the admitting office.

"She'd like to talk to you about the hospital. I think she's confused about the arrangements."

He called. I could hear their conversation. I could tell it wasn't she who was confused about the arrangements. I was the confused one.

He sat down in the chair opposite me. He was very solemn.

"Sally, the reason for being hospitalized is for us to do this work in the safest possible environment. That does mean that you wouldn't be able to leave the ward until I believe it's safe."

I was having a visceral response. Slightly out of body. But everything feeling very real. *This is happening. I've got to figure this out.* I believe what I was experiencing in this moment was my window of tolerance getting ready to explode, throwing me into chaos—and me working, mustering as much courage as possible not to be locked in rigidity.

I was looking for balance.

"How will that work?"

I don't think he was expecting this to be so hard for me.

"You would be on a floor..."

...with other people?

I guess I'd had visions of a private room, like when I'd had surgery a few years earlier. Lots of visitors and flowers.

His voice solemn. "Yes."

Really hard to take in.

Tears.

More tears.

I felt afraid. I felt as if I were disconnecting from the world. It felt like I'd be leaving forever. Like I'd never see Sam again.

"Sally—this will be a temporary arrangement."

"Are you sure?"

"Yes. It's important for me to get you somewhere safe to work on what's happening. We've no real idea what's going on and there are some warning signs I must pay attention to. It's a voluntary admittance. You can't leave the floor on your own—I'd have to give you permission. I'll be in charge, not the hospital. And I'll see you once or twice every day for therapy there. We'll do whatever it takes."

That was a little better.

I trusted him.

The fear of never getting out—being trapped—I'm sure was at least partially implicit. But as Dr. Siegel and I had discussed many times, that was the fear of a little girl with no advocates or agency. And I was a grown woman now, not a child. I also knew, when I thought it through, that Dr. Siegel would never trap me or trick me. He would keep me safe and advocate on my behalf. He always listened to me. I trusted him. At the end of it, I felt a little better, but I was still afraid.

"You know what, Sally?"

"What?"

"I have an idea. Give me a few hours—I'll get back to you soon."

LATER THAT EVENING, Dr. Siegel called to tell me what he had figured out.

"I have a plan. I think you'll be very comfortable with it."

I was to check in at UCLA in two days. Paul would take me; Dr. Siegel would meet me there. I arranged for our babysitter to be available to help Paul for as long as I was in the hospital. I explained to Sam that I'd be away for a while.

"Mommy will call you every day!"

I let my closest friends know, too. "I'll be gone a week—maybe a little longer. Don't worry! I'm in good hands—I just have some therapeutic work to do, and I need to be away from home to do it."

Again, I'm not sure anyone really understood. My closest friends knew I was in therapy for childhood abuse, but I hadn't shared my diagnosis; I don't believe that would have been helpful for anyone. MPD was mostly known then from movies that really didn't portray it in any way like my experience. Looking back now, those misguided films were a real hurdle for me.

I spent the next day hanging out with Sam. Paul and I avoided talking about it. All my emotional energy was working staying grounded with Sam. I just didn't know how to express what I was going through to Paul, and he let me know he was fine.

The next morning, I kissed Sammy goodbye. Huge hug. Told him how much I loved him. Our babysitter was there, and he loved her. Everything was in place.

I'll see you soon, Sammy.

I started crying the minute we drove away from the house.

At the hospital I asked Paul just to drop me off. I was trying to stop crying and knew it would be harder with him by my side. I think he was relieved.

I had to be buzzed into the door at the entrance to the unit I was being admitted to. The door swung shut and locked automatically behind me.

I was on the locked unit.

The nurse was expecting me and took me to a meeting room, right across from the nurses' station, where they'd check me in as soon as Dr. Siegel arrived. Feeling somewhere between Just Blank and No-Body, it was the first time I remember thinking, *Oh, this is what it was like to be me as a little kid*—present, but watching what was happening, more than being a part of it.

When I saw Dr. Siegel walking into the meeting room, I realized that since I'd started therapy, I hadn't seen him anywhere outside of his office. It added another layer of complexity to my experience. All the staff knew him and greeted him. I also hadn't been in a room with him and anyone else except Sam and Paul. I was feeling invisible until he greeted me. Once he had, I thought, *Okay. I'm here.* Grounded.

I don't know if Dr. Siegel had information I simply hadn't known, or if it was just a coincidence, but it would turn out to be a stroke of genius that in my early forties, as the mother of a young son, I was being admitted to the adolescent psychiatric unit at UCLA Medical Center.

Just me, the staff, and ten adolescent girls being treated for eating disorders.

It would turn out to be exactly where I belonged. Precisely what I needed.

It's my job to keep you safe, Sally.

And it soon became clear he was working overtime.

Brilliant.

AS THE NURSE AND ADMITTING PEOPLE were asking me questions, explaining the protocols and unit rules, Dr. Siegel was signing papers and discussing my care orders with them. The nurse who was ticking off questions from a checklist asked,

"Do you smoke?"

I wasn't expecting that. It threw me a little. And I kind of whispered,

"Um...yes."

Dr. Siegel turned his head toward me, looking puzzled. "You smoke?"

I hadn't smoked since my twenties. Over the last couple weeks, I'd smoked a couple of cigarettes with a friend and a neighbor who still smoked. We laughed as we snuck a smoke in here and there—feeling like kids again, hiding from the adults, except now we were adults hiding from the kids! I'd had a feeling I was going to want to smoke in the hospital, too, so I brought a pack with me. Paul didn't know, and I'd been careful not to let Sam know. I hadn't mentioned it to Dr. Siegel.

Busted.

"A little."

"Since when?"

"The last couple of weeks."

The nurse told him that as an adolescent floor, they required a parent or doctor's permission to allow me to smoke. Dr. Siegel and I shared a glance and a small laugh. For a minute I thought he might not sign the permission slip. I don't think he felt so good about it, but after hesitating, he signed. I was asked to turn my cigarettes and matches over to the nurse's station.

"Okay. They're in my bag. Shall I get them now?"

"No, we'll collect them when we go through your bag. We'll keep them for you at our station."

Go through my bag?

It was certainly a strange place to be. That my fellow patients were all adolescent girls took the edge off somehow. I had my own room and bathroom, but we shared a communal shower. Dr. Siegel left after we set a late afternoon time for our first session. A nurse showed me to my room. I had a small suitcase, and she went through everything piece by piece. She took my cuticle scissors and tweezers—no "sharps" allowed.

Next: a physical examination, another thing I wasn't expecting. It seemed the main purpose was to check for any cutting or other evidence of bodily harm. The doctor asked about the marks on my arm and foot, which were all mostly healed. I told him exactly what I'd done. Let him know that Dr. Siegel knew about it. He looked at my ears—I had not mentioned them because at Dr. Siegel's request, I had seen my doctor earlier to have them checked after the stabbing-stick news. Miraculously, no damage detected.

I retreated to my room. Decided to skip lunch so I could spend time getting my room set up. Arranged all the photos I'd brought of Sam on the ledge by my twin bed, and my drawing materials, books, and journals on a nearby shelf. As I was looking at the photos and journaling, I noticed the sliding peephole on the door that would allow the nurses to check in on me.

I was feeling on the verge of something. Suddenly I couldn't keep my eyes open. I lay down to take a nap.

WHEN THE NURSE CAME IN MY ROOM to tell me Dr. Siegel was there for our appointment, I woke up and immediately felt as disoriented as I ever had. It took a couple of minutes to understand who she was and what she was saying. It seemed I'd fallen into a deep, sound sleep. Groggy. Hazy. My body heavy and in slow motion. I knew where I was, but I was confused about it. As if I were coming out of a bad dream. Yet I had no recollection of dreaming.

"Thank you. I'll be right out."

I got myself together and went to meet him. He was in the room where I'd been taken for the admissions process. There were windows all around, so Dr. Siegel had closed the curtains for privacy, and it was a little dark. I felt nervous. He asked me how I was doing.

"Okay."

"You sure about that?"

"What do you mean?"

He was looking at me and I wasn't sure he knew it was me. His face looked a little worried.

I just started crying. Quiet tears.

"What's going on?"

I sat there for a long time. Speechless. No words. My eyes mostly closed, open just enough to see him, because I needed to know he was there.

"I'm not sure."

It felt like my body was as still as anyone could be. Barely breathing. Couldn't detect much of a heartbeat. Frozen.

"I feel crazy. I know I'm not. But it feels like maybe I am. I feel confused."

"Well, tell me a little more. Do you know how long you've been here?"

"Since this morning."

"How'd you get here?"

"Paul."

"Do you remember seeing me earlier?"

It was comforting to have him to check in with me like that.

"Uh-huh. I know where I am, Dr. Siegel. I just feel...feel...I feel otherworldly."

"Can you tell me more about that?"

"It's hard to say."

"What makes it hard to say?"

"The word that keeps coming up is 'labyrinth.'"

"What does that mean to you?"

That I'm just completely fucked up.

"When I close my eyes—when I look inside, I get confused. I don't know which way to go—where to look for or find any answers."

"That does sound confusing. Even scary."

"Yes, it is. I guess 'labyrinth' is just a fancy word for lost."

"Or maybe not so much lost, but on a path to find your way out. Which can be confusing, as you say. How does that feel to you?"

That sounded about right. A path out. I loved that Dr. Siegel was always so optimistic. He never doubted I would resolve the trauma of my childhood, that I'd dissolve the memory barriers of MPD, allowing me to recover from living a dissociated life.

How does it feel?

I think I must've had a scrunched-up face, eyes shut. Like a little kid thinking *If I can't see you, you can't see me.* Breathing suddenly heavier. Faster. On the verge of hyperventilating. I felt panicked.

"I'm afraid." I could barely get the words out of my mouth.

"Try taking some breaths, Sally. Slow, intentional breaths..."

Breathing in...breathing out...

"That's right. Try to keep your focus on your breath."

Focusing.

"Can you try opening your eyes?"

Eyes open.

"Try looking at me."

That helped. Seeing him there felt safe.

"I think it's better."

"Good."

A little time passed. It kept getting better.

Whew.

"Okay?"

"Better. That was scary."

He asked me to keep my eyes open, take a look around.

"I think you were on the verge of a panic attack. How's it now?"

On the verge.

"It feels strange."

"This is a new place for you. It's the hospital. I'd like to tell you something."

"What's that?"

He told me he'd trained on this floor and was the director of this very unit not so long ago.

"I know and have worked with the staff. They're going to take good care of you while we do our work. You're safe here."

"It feels safest to you for me to be here?"

"Yes, it does. I think it's the safest place for you right now. And the safest place for you and me to do our work."

"Okay. Good."

That feels better. Grounding.

"I just can't stop crying."

"Can you tell me about your tears?"

And just then, I realized I had indeed been dreaming during my nap. "Right before you got here for our appointment, I was napping, and I had a nightmare. Can you have a nightmare during a nap?"

"I believe you can."

"I think I did."

"Did you write about it in your journal?"

"Not yet—I'm only just remembering it."

"Will it help to tell me about it?"

"Remember when I first walked in here, you asked me if I knew who you were?"

"Yes."

"Why did you ask me that?"

"When I first saw you, I wasn't sure you knew me. You looked confused when you came in—so I was checking in with you."

"I did know who you were."

"You did. You said my name."

"The thing is—I don't think I knew who *I* was."

I leaned back and closed my eyes. I was still crying, still feeling groggy. My body felt heavy.

"Can you tell me about your nightmare?"

I took a momentary dive inside and then came back up. It took me a little while to gather my thoughts. I knew what I'd dreamt but I had to make sure I had it right. It gave me a sad feeling. Very sad.

"I was afraid I was dead, Dr. Siegel. I woke up and I thought I'd died."

I opened my eyes and saw his face. He just looked at me with real concern.

"I died in my dream."

"Tell me what that was like for you."

I started crying more. Not quiet tears, but not really loud either. Pain-filled tears. I was feeling a depth of pain I hadn't really known before.

"It just hurts so bad, Dr. Siegel. I feel like I'm in a lot of trouble here."

"Tell me what is hurting so bad, Sally."

"Don't let anything happen to me."

"I won't. The staff will take good care of you. They can call me if anything happens. That is why we decided to come here—remember—to keep you safe."

"I remember."

"Can you tell me what has you so worried? What you're afraid might happen?"

"I'm so afraid..."

I couldn't say it. I just cried for a while. He just listened to my sobs.

Okay. I could say it. What I was so afraid of. What my tears were all about. All I could think about was...

"I don't want Sam to lose me." I didn't understand where this terror was coming from.

We finished our session and Dr. Siegel left. We planned to meet early the next afternoon. I went to lie down and was still crying, so hard the nurse came to check on me. My face was swollen and red all over from the tears and from the hundreds of scratchy hospital tissues

I was using to wipe them all away. I washed my face. All I wanted to do was sleep.

Next thing I knew, a nurse was there to tell me it was dinner time. I asked if I could eat in my room—I was so upset I didn't want the other patients to see me like this. She understood but said that was against policy. I could eat in the room where I'd met with Dr. Siegel, but the curtains would have to remain open, and she'd have to sit with me. As it turned out, I couldn't eat a thing. I think that set off some red flags—it was a unit treating young girls with eating disorders, after all. But either they called Dr. Siegel or decided on their own that it was okay for me to skip dinner.

I WAS EXHAUSTED. I couldn't read, draw, or journal. I was just too tired and scattered. I wanted to call home. I went to where the phones were, and other patients were in line, so I waited for my turn. It was the first time I was with the other patients. They were friendly but had no idea who I was or what I was doing there. And I was so disoriented and upset I could barely speak. But I did my best to respond to their greetings. When it was my turn at the phone, I spoke only briefly to Paul because it took so much effort not to sound upset or to cry. When he asked how I was, I think I told him I was having a hard time, but I was fine. I'd seen Dr. Siegel and would see him again tomorrow.

"Okay Sally—take care. Don't worry about us—Sam's fine. We'll talk tomorrow. Love you."

"Love you."

"Here's Sammy."

"Where are you, Mommy?"

"I'm at my meeting." It's what I'd told him about going away—that I had to be at some meetings.

"I love you, Mommy."

"I love you, Sam. Big kiss. Sleep tight, sweetie. Talk tomorrow."

I couldn't keep the tears from gushing. I just couldn't stop. When I got back to my room and saw all the photos of Sam I began sobbing uncontrollably. Soon the nurse came in to check on me and when she saw Sam's photos, she asked about him. I told her about adopting him in Romania. How I'd never left him overnight.

"How was your call with him?"

"It was good. Sweet. He's fine. He's home with his dad."

The nurse was so thoughtful and caring. She calmed me down some.

But not for long.

It was an incredibly painful night. Life-stealing pain. My tears wouldn't stop. I didn't know it was possible to cry for that length of time. It was difficult to breathe. My face was a mess, raw, and the tissues were not helping.

I fell in and out of sleep all night. I could hear the nurses peeking in to check on me. I was pray, pray, praying for sleep.

Crying myself to sleep.

Burning tears.

Full-body pain.

I was inconsolable.

WHEN MY EYES OPENED, I knew where I was, but I wasn't sure why. First thing I noticed were Sam's photos. A deeply felt sense of longing. Longing and loss. Loss and longing—painful. I did know that Sam was safe. But I had so many feelings and awarenesses swirling around within at that moment that I couldn't really make out a clear thought. When the nurse checked in on me, that brought some clarity.

Oh right—I'm in the hospital because I need to be safe.

I noticed I was curled up in a fetal position.

Hope, hope, hoping they served coffee in the UCLA hospital adolescent psychiatric unit.

I went to the dining room and grabbed a coffee. Most of the girls were there. They were living with lots of food rules. Very measured portions. They had minders, I learned, who watched them for some time after each meal to ensure no one could purge. They were all so very thin. I learned many of them had been here for lengthy stays, having been transferred from medical units where in some cases they'd been fighting for their lives.

Fighting for their lives.

Was I fighting for mine?

I took my coffee, got my cigarettes from the nurse's station, and went for a smoke in the smoking room. The room was all windows facing into the unit. There I was, smoking. Eight-thirty in the morning. I could see some of the girls looking my way. Did they think I was stupid for smoking? At that hour? In that place? An adult in their psych ward? Or were they wishing they could smoke too, but their parents wouldn't sign the permission slip? *This must've been what it was like to be me as a teenager,* I thought. *Smoking and not even liking it. Thinking it was just what I was supposed to do.* Such a confusing time. I put the cigarette out and went back to my room.

I wanted to check my journal to see if out of all the painful and deep emotional crying, any states had written in the Bulletin Board. Any smokers in the group? There was nothing. Everything within felt shut down. I thought about sketching, but nothing came. Though I was not crying now, my eyes were too sore, red, and swollen from yesterday to read. So, I just sat there. Looking out the window in my room. It was near where the hospital helicopters landed on the roof, and I could hear them coming in and taking off. Coming in and taking off. Taking off. Taking off. Within me there was a confused desire to do the same.

Please, please, can I just get out of here.

I decided to sleep until I could see Dr. Siegel.

WHEN DR. SIEGEL ARRIVED, he let me know the only room available for us to work in that day was a padded room.

Really? Padded room?

I think I must've closed my eyes immediately and tears started trickling down my face. I looked inside and then opened my eyes to say,

"That seems like it might actually be a good idea."

"Why's that?"

"Is it soundproof too?"

"Yes."

"I have this feeling I may need to scream."

We walked down a hall, then came to a heavy door with a small square window, kind of like the door to my room, only it was covered from the inside. We walked in. Padded walls. No chairs. We sat on the floor. My face, my head, and my mind were all a mess.

Dr. Siegel left for a moment and came back with some pillows. As we settled in, he let me know he'd been in touch with the nurses last night and this morning.

"I understand you had a difficult night."

"I did."

"What's going on?"

It took me quite some time to collect my thoughts enough to be able to speak.

"Feels like I'm weaving in and out of consciousness...having trouble staying grounded. I keep wanting to close my eyes and go to sleep, but then I can't."

"What's keeping you from sleeping?"

"It's just a bombardment of thoughts, fears, flashes, ideas, longings, needs, feelings, emotions...I can't hold on to anything long enough to know what it is."

"The nurses let me know you were crying heavily much of the night."

"I mean, look at my face."

"Yes—I see."

His face exuded compassion. For me. I always felt like he could feel what I was feeling—not taking it away for me or protecting me from it, simply being there with me with it. Widening, widening windows every step of the way.

"Do you know what the tears are about?"

Sitting there on the floor, my head leaning against the padded wall, working on catching a whole thought. Took some time.

"I used to hardly ever cry, Dr. Siegel. Do you remember me telling you when we first started working together—I can't remember why I said it, what we were talking about—but I said, very proudly, that I had a very high tolerance for pain. Like—'Yay! It's a good thing.' Do you remember me saying that?"

"Yes, I remember that."

"Do you remember what you said to me?"

"Remind me."

"You said, very gently and kindly, you weren't so sure that was a good thing."

"Yes. I do remember. What was it like for you to hear me say that?"

Oh wow. "Like so many things back then, I was stunned by your answer. Not stunned that you said it but stunned when I really thought about it...oh my god—high tolerance for pain—not such a great thing, unless you're being tortured. So, go figure, you know."

"Go figure what?"

"I *was* being tortured. I don't know, Dr. Siegel—maybe I'm crying so much now because I could never cry then."

"What would happen when you cried then?"

"Tortured," I said. And it was true. I'd be punished.

It didn't feel strange to be sitting in a padded room anymore. With him there with me, resonating with my pain, I felt safe. And I knew I could dive to even deeper depths to figure out what was going on.

"I know there's more...It scares me."

"Please tell me about 'more.' More of what?"

"It feels like there's a war inside. And even though I know I'm safe here with you—it *feels* dangerous. Whatever's about to happen feels dangerous."

"To look deeper inside?"

"It feels like there's one state that's fighting to be known. And it feels dangerous...destructive."

Dr. Siegel sat with that a little bit, and then reminded me about the feeling of impending danger.

"You mean about it being implicit—the memory of how childhood felt. Childhood being dangerous, not dangerous to remember?"

"Yes—as a possibility," Dr. Siegel confirmed. "That you're safe here with me. I feel I'm safe."

Hospital.

Padded room.

"Right. It's hard for me sometimes to hold on to that."

"How about if I invite this state to come, with safety precautions?"

"Okay. I don't know if I can stay for it—but I'll try."

"What makes it hard for you to stay?"

"I have this feeling it's explosive. It's mean."

"It might be helpful to let that state express itself. Remember—mad is different than rage."

"Okay—so maybe just mad, not explosive."

"Maybe."

"There's this feeling that's been haunting me—and I think it's this state. It's really mad."

"At whom?"

"Me. At all the states."

"Well, shall we give this state the opportunity to let us know what's going on?"

An opportunity. Yes, an opportunity to learn more. That helped.

"All right. Just give me a minute, okay?"

I closed my eyes, trying to bring up the feelings that had haunted me much of the night. The fear. I was working on sitting with the idea of such an angry or explosive state. On accepting that it's okay to be mad.

"I guess, Dr. Siegel, I'm afraid to know everything—but I'm working on widening that window."

"Wonderful."

"Before you send out the invitation—can I ask you something?"

"Ask me anything you'd like."

"Part of my hesitation is this feeling that the other states don't know about this state, and it might cause a bunch of confusion."

"I understand that."

"If I'm able to widen my window—will the other states' windows widen automatically?"

"Well, that's a great question. My hope is for all states to widen the window of tolerance for knowing what happened. I think inviting this state you feel wants to come talk will help us get closer to that."

"Okay. Give me a minute."

"Take your time."

I stretched out on the floor with my head on a pillow. But I just couldn't get comfortable. I sat up, moved the pillow behind my back against the padded wall, and took another pillow and held it in my lap.

Protection.

Took some breaths.

"Ready."

Dr. Siegel sent out the invitation. The arrival of this state seemed to take longer than any of the others. And when it came, it was actually quiet. Not what I was expecting.

"I'm not going to hurt anyone. Why's everyone so worried about me?"

Maybe not so dangerous.

"Welcome."

"Thank you. You're Dr. Siegel?"

"I am. May I know your name?"

"Jessica."

"Jessica—thank you for coming. Can you tell me when you were born?"

"Fourteen."

"And what was your purpose?"

"To be alive. To have a good time. To have friends."

To be a fucking teenager.

"Those are all great purposes."

"Yes! Thank you. They made it so hard for me."

"Who?"

"The little girls."

"How did they make it hard for you?"

"Because I was alive. And liked to have fun. Friends. They hated that."

"Why did they hate that?"

"Because being alive and noticed wasn't safe in that house or that body. So, they all just sat around being quiet. I hate that. Which is why I've got to get out of this fucking body. Oh, sorry."

"Why are you sorry?"

"Saying 'fucking.'"

"Why is that bad?"

"Because anything that brings attention feels dangerous to them. And that's why I want to get rid of them. They just want me to stay quiet."

"And what brings attention?"

"Everything."

"Everything?"

"And anything."

"I'm not quite sure I follow?"

"Being a little kid in that house, Dr. Siegel. That's what was dangerous. Not me. It was dangerous just breathing. Saying good morning. Eating. Playing. Sleeping. Being alive."

"I see. Just being them."

"And being little."

"Was dangerous."

"Yes."

"How would getting rid of them help you?"

"Then it can just be me. I'm ready for it to be just my body and not have to share it anymore."

"Can you tell me about taking over the body? How do you plan to do that?"

"I can't tell you that."

"Why not?"

"Because then you'll want to get rid of me."

"No...oh no...I have no wish to get rid of you. I'd like to help you. I'd like to understand why you want to get rid of them and have the body to yourself. Letting me know how you want to do that will help me help you."

"Well, I'm just tired of them—tired of how they are, and tired of how Sally can't know anything."

"What are the things Sally can't know?"

"Oh, fuck."

"What?"

"No one wants to hear about this from me."

"I'd like to hear it."

"What about Sally?"

"Can you ask her?"

"Let's ask her together."

"Wouldn't it be easier just to get rid of her?"

"Can you tell me how you'd get rid of her?"

There was quite a long silence...and then Jessica let Dr. Siegel and me know that it was she who wanted me to drive off the Coast Highway. I got the feeling it was more of a wish than a command or intention. And I think she was saying she wanted to get rid of me, not kill me. She wanted me out of the way, not dead. It occurred to me that perhaps Jessica was mean the way eighth-grade mean girls are mean. She was a kid. Not so dangerous. Teenager dangerous. Mostly frustrated and frustrating.

Consequences were not her strong suit.

I was feeling safer.

Dr. Siegel thanked her for letting him know all this. He checked in with me to see how I was. I told him I was fine.

Then he talked to her about the body.

"Do you know that you're not separate from Sally or any of the states?"

"That's what I want to fix."

"I understand that. But you all are part of one body."

"I want the body to be just mine."

Dr. Siegel went on to let her know if she got rid of me, or any of the other states, by hurting the body, the body would be gone too. That Jessica was part of a system my mind created to keep me safe.

"Can you tell me what life has been like for you?"

"I hate being part of that family. I want it to be just me. Just me in the body. And no fucking parents."

"I think I might be coming to understand what you're going through."

"I doubt it."

"Can you tell me?"

"You know how Sally can't say 'sex'?"

"Yes. Is Sally listening?"

I let them know I was. It was okay.

"She can't say it because of what the mother did."

"Did to who?"

"To every state! Well—to the little girls."

"What did she do?"

"SEX!!!"

I was quiet. Tears streaming.

"She made them all so sexual that I could never be. They made it impossible. I just wanted to be a normal teenager. All I wanted was to have a boyfriend. I wanted to be like my friends. But she made sex so fucked up. She ruined it for me. And Sally's father, too. I hate that all those fucking feelings come from them."

I knew what she meant. I wished it too. I wished that all those sexual feelings could've been mine, and mine alone. I wished they could've been memories of making love the first time with someone I really cared about and who cared about me. I so deeply wished that those feelings wouldn't have been reminders of childhood. Of sexual abuse from my parents.

That would've been so perfect.

Jessica's memories broke my heart.

"All I wanted was a boyfriend."

I knew that feeling.

I suddenly had a flash of me, in high school, sitting in the back of my boyfriend's van. I was sixteen so he would've been seventeen. I liked him so much. He really liked me. I loved when we kissed. It wasn't just a crush—there was a genuine connection. I wanted to be with him so badly. I wanted him to be the first person I had sex with. We were making out, but I was starting to feel like I was suffocating. It was so hot. He wasn't doing anything wrong, but when I told him I couldn't stand being that close—it felt like I couldn't breathe—I mean the look he gave me was—well, to this day, it makes me sad. So sad. I couldn't have sex then. Everything that happened to me in that family just got in the way.

I was beginning to know what Jessica was talking about. Beginning to remember things. How anything sexual for me, at that time in my life, was horrifying. And not horrifying because it was bad or painful or dangerous with the boy I so wanted to be with. But horrifying and bad and painful and dangerous because anything sexual for me at sixteen was a minefield.

And it was Jessica's job to walk through that minefield without getting blown up.

No wonder she wanted to get rid of me.

She wasn't explosive. My parents were. Always an explosion from them.

Dr. Siegel asked Jessica if she could tell him more about what happened.

Jessica hated me, my mother, and all the little girl states who were sexualized by my mother. What she did was abusive and terribly brutal, mad, and twisted. Yes, crazy. Arousing little girls so that they were always wanting to masturbate. Always wanting to be close to her. Some even seeking her out to be sexual. To get that feeling. And then the feeling would get them in trouble. She would hurt them. Sometimes for having that feeling. Sometimes for not having that feeling. She would make them lie on the green blanket on her bed and do things to them. The noises. The sounds. The smell. All things that were haunting me now. And Jessica hated them for liking the feelings.

There were so many states to protect me from the feelings, so I didn't have to know the feelings. But then I couldn't have any feelings. And there was still a part of me that wanted to have the normal feelings—to be a normal teenager and have a boyfriend. That was Jessica.

The entire time Jessica was explaining all this, I was getting flashes of pain all over my body. I recognized them as flashbacks. Intrusive. Implicit. I realized too what Dr. Siegel had meant when he'd said that something bad was not *going* to happen. Something bad had *already* happened. Something bad always happened then.

All the time.

There was no safety there.

But I survived it. I've already survived.

There was safety here.

Dr. Siegel explained to Jessica how it wasn't the little girls' fault. Bodies—even little bodies—are hardwired to feel sexual. It was the mother who was at fault. Not the little girls.

By this point, as we neared the end of the session, I was so exhausted. Dr. Siegel too. He wanted to talk to Jessica about one more thing, though, before we wrapped up for the day.

"I'd like you to tell me about wanting to have Sally drive off the highway."

"I just thought it would help me. I see now that it wouldn't have."

"Do you know why Sally didn't drive off the road?"

"No. Do I have to?"

"I think it might be important for her to tell you and for you to hear it."

"Does she want to tell me?"

"Shall we ask her?"

"Okay."

I let Jessica know the reason I didn't drive off the coast highway was because I don't want to die.

"Why not? Why not—your life's so boring."

Mean-girl mean.

The tears came so fast.

"I don't want to die because I love my son very much and don't want him to lose me. I want him to have a better childhood than I did. Better than we did. I want him to have a better mother than I did."

I want to be a better mother.

There was a very long silence. Very, very quiet.

Finally, Jessica acknowledged that she hadn't thought about Sam. She hadn't thought about me being a mother—or that a mother could be good, or that it could be good to be a mother or have a mother. I think the idea of anyone wanting to be a mother was too much for her to take in.

Dr. Siegel wanted her to know that all mothers aren't bad. Not all mothers hurt their children. Or have sex with them.

"That mother is a monster," Jessica said.

"She was," Dr. Siegel agreed.

"Do you know the worst thing she'd do to them, Dr. Siegel?"

"No. What's the worst thing she'd do to them?"

Oh no, oh no, oh no.

I knew.

"She'd bite them."

Sending electrical currents of pain through my whole body.

Zapppppp........Zappppppppp.......Zappppppppp.....Zappppppppp...

"Where'd she bite them?"

This was all beginning to sink in for me. My mother would bite. She would bite my vagina. I was just a little girl. If what she was doing made me feel good, she'd bite me. If what she was doing hurt, she'd bite me. She would bite my vagina. All the sad little girls I drew were crying from the pain she inflicted.

Sadistic fucking monster.

I kind of always knew it. Knew something wasn't right. For so long I'd wished it wasn't true. I never wanted it to be true. But it was true. Now I really knew it.

I had the answer to "What kind of childhood did you have?"

It was a sexual childhood. It was all about sex. There. I said it. Sex.

Fuck them.

I thought it was great how Jessica kept saying fuck.

"Jessica, I fucking love how you fucking say fuck."

Evil fucking mother monster.

I fucking hate her more than ever.

The energy I was so afraid of with Jessica...it was exploding within me...inside out...

It was my energy.

My explosion.

Then I screamed.

Out loud.

At first into the pillow.

Really loud.

Then I remembered. Padded room. Soundproof.

I just let it out.

"I FUCKING HATE HER!!"

I was crying so hard.

Loudly.

I was inconsolable.

But now I knew why.

OVER THE NEXT TWO DAYS, more and more unfolded.

Jessica hated how everything that happened to the little girls had ruined her ability to have a normal life like her friends. Having a boyfriend was out of the question, because sex was either something that made us freeze, go into a panic, pass out, or just want more and more. She was so aware of all of those states, and she couldn't risk being sexual with anyone ever. And she hated the mother for doing that, and she hated the little girls who were sexual. She hated that she was the only girl at fourteen who was not a virgin, like all her friends talked about. She hated that the most. She could never talk to anyone about sex because it was so confusing. And the feelings were always with her. As for me, I had kept that all secret, and she was angry at me about that.

"Why didn't you ever say anything?" she asked me, in the padded room.

"She was hurting me too. The way I protected myself from knowing and feeling the pain of it all was to divide up. All the little girls kept me safe. I'm sorry I couldn't do more. But I'm glad I survived. I'm glad to know about you now. I'm glad you did your part. I'm glad we are all here making sense of what was so insane."

I'm glad you all played your parts so well.

I was remembering more about how all I wanted in high school was a boyfriend. In college too. There were a few that I really wanted to have a relationship with. I couldn't. It was always too dangerous. Too humiliating. Shame-filled. Sad. Very sad. Whenever I got that close to a boy, I felt like I might die. Painful.

"I'm sorry, Jessica. I'm sorry about it all."

Very carefully and compassionately, Dr. Siegel had opened the lines of communication between me and all my states. I was beginning to know my childhood, what had happened to me. The divided, fragmented states were showing me the big picture as the memory barriers between states were dissolving. I was no longer needing them. The states were beginning to communicate internally and with me and Dr. Siegel. I was beginning to have an awareness of how Dr. Siegel described integration—"it's the linkage of differentiated states, Sally."

Memory barriers were becoming less rigid, *and* less chaotic.

This was a significant step toward my healing.

"It's not really possible to make sense of your mother and father's behavior and abuse," Dr. Siegel told me. "But it is possible to begin to make sense of the impact it had on you...for years."

What it means to me now.

Jessica no longer wanted to get rid of me. She was relieved to know that Sam had a good mom. She came to understand that there was only one body. With my help and with Jennifer's, Dr. Siegel was able to get us communicating in ways that were helpful. Compassionate. Not harmful. We were able to help Jessica begin to grieve the loss of all the things an adolescent was meant to experience as only an adolescent can. I think it helped when Jessica realized it was my loss as well. It was a loss I'd always had an inkling of, just not so clearly as now.

Going into the hospital I was so afraid I was having a nervous breakdown. Now, as I was preparing to go home, I could see it was as Dr. Siegel had described—a breakthrough.

I spent not quite a full week at the hospital. On my last morning before checking out, I ate breakfast with the girls on the unit. And I joined them in the lounge after. Sitting there with ten teenage girls seemed like perfect timing to me. They were great company. They certainly had challenges to face; they no doubt had their own stories to make sense of. They were curious about my presence among them, and I let them know the truth—I'd been there to do some intensive work on some things with my therapist.

"Did it work?" one of them asked.

"It's working—I still have a way to go. It takes time."

They seemed to understand what I meant.

They ranged in age from around fourteen to eighteen. They were fun and funny. Interesting. Sad and worried. Trying to figure things out. The next day some of them were expecting visits from their parents, and a few of them didn't seem to be looking forward to it. They seemed to feel misunderstood by their parents.

Mostly though, they talked about their boyfriends.

And said "fuck" a lot.

When I went back to my room to gather my things, I found I was grateful that I hadn't had to go back and forth between Dr. Siegel's office and home all these days. As much as I'd missed Sam and Paul, I knew I had needed this time in the hospital to do the work I'd just done. My thoughts were much clearer now.

I stopped at the nurses' station to thank them and asked them to throw my cigarettes away.

As I left the locked unit to meet Paul downstairs to drive home, I was hoping the girls on the floor had therapists as good as mine.

PART 3

IN THE CAR, PAUL said he could tell something positive had happened in the hospital. "You look really good, Sally—more relaxed than in a while."

He was curious about what my experience had been.

"It was intense, Paul. I know a lot more now about what childhood was like for me. It was painful and disturbing..." I needed to pause and take a breath. It was never easy to talk about what happened in therapy—it was so private for me—but I wanted to answer him... "But I'm grateful to know it now."

He looked at me, caringly, acknowledging my pain. I think it reflected how painful this all was for him, too. It was hard for us both.

"Can you tell me about what you and Dr. Siegel figured out?"

I took another breath, and closed my eyes, looking inside, and then answered him—eyes open.

"I'm understanding more about how my diagnosis works—not so much that I have different parts, but that I have many states of mind that faced and protected me. From unspeakable things, Paul...What my parents did was...well, just horrific."

That was as much as I wanted to say. It's not that I *couldn't* share the details of the padded room with him—it was that I didn't need to. Bringing that into my life with him and Sam was not what I wanted. Keeping therapy separate from my home life felt right. Right for the three of us. I wasn't just being protective of me—but also of Sam and Paul. And just as I didn't feel the need to share the complexities of

134

therapy, Paul didn't feel a need to hear them. It wasn't a secret. It was private. He respected that. What we shared in this moment was less of the details and more of the feeling. He was aware of the emotional impact my time in the hospital had on me, attuned to it, and I was so relieved he could see how good it had been for me.

"I could never have done the work I did outside of the hospital. Thank you, Paul, for being so supportive."

"I'm very happy to see you've gotten some answers. It's good you went."

He reached for my hand.

"I love you, Sally."

"I love you too, Paul."

ARRIVING HOME WAS WONDERFUL. Sam was happy to see me. I was happy to be home.

The three of us took a long walk on the beach with the dogs. It was grounding to have my feet in the sand and the water...throwing tennis balls for the dogs. We were all laughing. At the heart of it, I realized I was a happy person. That despite everything, I'd made myself a good life. It was good to know that out of excruciating pain had come so much clarity.

It wasn't all positive, what I felt as I walked along the beach. I was also noticing some intrusive thoughts. Feelings. Remembering some of the things Jessica had revealed. About Little Sally. Dead mom. Green blanket. Vomit. And when I remembered the vomit, I wasn't feeling sick to my stomach any longer, but my whole body would feel a jolt from the inside out. I was also remembering some things that just seemed random. The sexual things. The sexual things felt rapid-fire and made me dizzy...but they didn't make me feel sick anymore, not like they'd used to. It was different since the hospital and the padded room. They were different.

I realized that the sensations were different because now, I understood precisely where they came from. I knew the truth.

As I walked along the beach, I realized that along with the knowledge I'd gained, after the hospital, there was a great sense of grief. Full-body, hard-to-move grief. And it wasn't just feelings from childhood—it was grief for so much I'd lost because of my childhood. Everything Jessica had longed for. The deep emotional pain of the loss of all I had wished for.

Dr. Siegel and I would spend many months processing this complex set of feelings.

Things continued to be hard, but not prohibitively so. Hard, but not terrifying.

But in this moment, I was watching Sam, on his dad's shoulders, as they walked a little ahead of me—and I loved the sight of them. I felt safe. At the heart of my childhood, there'd been nothing resembling safety.

Nothing even close.

I was safe here.

Sam was safe here.

Sam had a safe childhood.

I was happy to be home.

I was happy.

I was beginning to wonder, where did happiness come from? Had I ever known a moment of happiness as a kid? Was there ever a moment that hadn't been contaminated by the horrific things happening to me in that family?

In the midst of so much cruelty, trauma, and massive unhappiness, how could I have ever been happy? And yet, I sensed that I had been. Somehow. How had I kept happiness alive? How could I feel it now?

Or was I happy only *because* of now?

Since I'd made a family of my own?

As hard as I tried, I couldn't recall a moment of happiness in the family I'd been born into.

At the end of that first weekend home after the hospital, a sense of sadness began to infiltrate my thoughts and feelings. Was it implicit memory of the sadness of my childhood that I was mistaking for sadness now? Or was it sadness now for all I'd just discovered? Sadness for all the states had endured?

Sadness for now, or then?

Perhaps both.

I just couldn't tell.

I was looking forward to talking to Dr. Siegel about it soon.

WHEN I GOT TO HIS OFFICE, he asked me how I was feeling.

"I feel different."

"Okay. Can you talk about different how?'

"When I got home—so happy to be home with Sam and Paul. And I have a deep sense of happiness about my life now. Somehow, I managed to keep that alive. But..."

"But what?"

"There's also this profound sense of sadness, Dr. Siegel."

"Ah—happy and sad."

"I can't figure out how I can know this feeling of happiness after everything I went through. And I can't figure out if the sadness is the sadness of childhood, or the sadness from knowing about my childhood. And does the happiness I know now have any roots in childhood? Are babies born happy? For that matter, can they be born sad?"

"These are such great questions. It's completely possible, Sally, to feel two opposite feelings at the same time."

I had to think for a moment. "I know I did, but—how could I have felt happy when I was a kid?"

"How do you know you did?"

"I feel it, at my innermost core. It's down deep. It had to be there."

I was really quiet for a bit. I started to cry.

"Tell me about your tears."

Two opposite feelings at the same time. "My tears, I think, Dr. Siegel, are tears of happiness—happiness to have survived—but they're also tears of sadness now for knowing what I went through—and for what I had to do to survive. What all the states had to do."

I was just really quiet, and then it occurred to me...

"Do you think in some way the states were created to protect my happiness?"

"Such a good question. Let's work on figuring that out."

Yes. A good question.

"You've just come off a very intense week at the hospital. How are you feeling about it now?"

I had to pause for a moment. There was something I wanted to say to him—and I was suddenly feeling so emotional. Having a hard time speaking, even, over the emotion that I was knowing, feeling, experiencing...everything in awareness at once.

"It was intense," I managed, at last.

I was trying to organize my thoughts. I so wanted to express to him what I was feeling.

"Thank you, Dr. Siegel. I'm so grateful for your help. Thank you for arranging the hospital like that. I'm feeling so much. And so much I'm feeling is awful because I know more. What my childhood was like. It hurts. It's painful. But it's different now. Not so terrifying as it was. I could never have done it without your help."

"You're so welcome, Sally. Thank you for doing the work you're doing."

"I don't know what I would've done if I hadn't met you." It was true. I might never have made sense of anything and lived in the mistaken fear that there was something wrong with Sam forever. And that would have been horrible—and not just for me, but for Sam.

"It's really good we met. It's a real honor, Sally, working with you."

I think he was taking in as much as I was. There was so much *to* take in.

"If I ask you a question," I said, "will you answer it?"

"Yes. Anything."

"What are you thinking about all this, Dr. Siegel?"

I was looking at him and he smiled. Almost chuckled. Took his time answering.

"I'm thinking how much courage you have. How brave you are to go right into making sense of things that are so difficult to know."

That made me smile.

And of course...his next question: "Can you tell me what that smile is about?"

"I'm smiling for so many reasons."

"Can you share one reason?"

I laughed. "Well, after knowing all I know from the hospital now, I'm smiling that I even know how to smile."

I went on to tell him more. That I was smiling because for the first time since we'd started therapy, I was beginning to know so much that I could imagine what was ahead. I knew there would be things that would be painful to know. To feel. Maybe even to smell, taste, and hear. I knew it would be hard...but not scary. Or scary, but not terrifying.

I knew what it was.

Mostly.

"How do you think you can know what's ahead and still smile, Sally?"

"Because now I know the terrible things happened a long time ago. I know they won't ever happen again."

"That's right, Sally. They already happened. Remembering is painful, not dangerous. Remembering, and differentiating what happened then from what's happening now, is integrative. That you're able to do it means you're becoming more and more free from the constraints of your childhood."

Free from the constraints.

The truth is my friend.

The truth will set me free.

I was not free yet, not all the way. But I was beginning to understand what "free" was.

And then kind of out of nowhere, my whole body felt a jolt. Dr. Siegel noticed. He looked at me, puzzled.

"What's going on, Sally?"

I was remembering something—something that had just come to me, in a flash. A flashback? But not like any flashback I'd ever experienced before.

"Dr. Siegel, can a flashback be of something good?"

"Tell me what you're feeling."

I told him I'd been remembering when I was a little kid—in DC, before I turned eight—when I could hear my dad's footsteps coming to my room...

It wasn't easy to say, but I *could* say it now, not just write it—

"...to be sexual with me. I would look out my window—which was right next to my bed—and I could see my tree."

"Your tree?"

"Yes."

I hadn't remembered it until now, yet it felt like something I had never forgotten...it was so vivid!

"The girl who lived across the street, who was nice to me—she was three years older, more my sister's friend—and there was a big willow tree in her family's yard and her dad gave her that tree..."

"I can clearly remember hearing her, so many years ago...'Daddy, can I have that tree? Can I have a hammock there?'

"Of course you can, Jennifer," her dad had said. "That's your tree!"

"Her name was Jennifer?" Dr. Siegel asked.

"It was," I said. I hadn't realized it myself until now. "Jennifer... wow...she was nice to me. Her parents were nice to me. They liked me. I always liked Jennifer. Wanted to be like her. She had a great laugh. Her parents had great laughs."

"I loved being over there. And Jennifer seemed so much smarter, like she knew stuff I didn't...like she could take care of herself. When I was at her house, no matter how many kids were over, she always knew everything and was in charge. I liked that about her."

Dr. Siegel noted the similarity to my Jennifer. I did too.

"Back to the tree. Your tree."

"So, I made the tree outside my window mine, too. And even if I couldn't see it because it was dark out...I knew it was there...and when I knew he was on his way...I could...I could..."

"You could what?"

"I could go 'poof'...and be in my tree."

"What happened in your tree?"

Magic.

Before I knew what I'd even said...I heard my voice say...

"Happy. Happiness happened in my tree."

The tree was where my happy memories were made. Where it was safe to have them, know them, and keep them safe. To be happy.

Safe.

Dr. Siegel said he didn't think that was a flashback.

"It sounds more like a memory, Sally. A good memory from your childhood."

A good memory.

No question...a breakthrough.

THE NEXT FEW MONTHS we worked a lot on processing what had happened in the padded room, and on happiness, sadness, and the tree. In one session, Dr. Siegel asked me to look inside and be curious about happiness. This is when we both first met the state named Peggy.

"Hi, Peggy."

"Hi, Dr. Siegel."

Peggy was born around my fifth birthday. Over many sessions, Peggy let Dr. Siegel and me know about how she kept happiness alive.

"With my dreams."

All I remembered ever having was nightmares.

"Not those kinds of dreams."

"What kind?"

I'm not sure if that was Dr. Siegel asking or me—at this point, we were all working together.

"The kind I made up."

Fantasies.

The way I hear it in my head now is that Dr. Siegel and I asked Peggy, together, "Can you tell us about that?" I imagine I was thinking it, he was asking it.

What transpired over a few sessions was Peggy's imagination, her fantasy of the life she imagined.

It started with President Kennedy.

My family lived in the suburbs of Washington DC when President Kennedy was elected. I remember my oldest sister being interested in politics and talking about him a lot. His picture was everywhere—in the papers, on TV. And I could remember—through Peggy—that I was mesmerized by the photographs of him and his little daughter. Smaller than me. They always looked happy. They looked magical. I remember something about Camelot and him and the soundtrack of that play that my oldest sister played all the time.

Peggy described how the fantasy went:

The family I lived in was the wrong family. Somehow I got stuck with them. President Kennedy was my real father, but he didn't know it yet. Once he figured it out, he would rescue me. But he would have to move heaven and earth to find me. Whenever he got close, I would run away and hide. Eventually, though, he would find me. And when he did, he would be my father. And I would be happy.

It was a happy I could feel. The feeling of safe...secure. Away from them.

Dr. Siegel wanted to be clear about who 'them' was.

Peggy made it clear she meant the family we were stuck in.

It was a feeling I knew. From then.

"Is it possible for happiness to be implicit?"

"I think so."

When I was eight years old, and we'd moved from DC to Chapel Hill, I was in class—fourth grade—when our teacher told us President Kennedy had been shot. He died.

But my fantasy did not die. It evolved. It always featured a famous, good father. He had to work hard to find me. And he did. I was always happy with him.

In some ways, the fantasies that started with Peggy became almost a road map for my life. It was like she was leaving breadcrumbs for me to follow, to get away from that family and find the life I had been dreaming of.

"I guess that was the whole point of fragmenting—of Peggy and the other states, of MPD—to keep me sane, to keep happy alive. To keep happy protected from crazy."

THERE WAS SOMETHING ELSE that was starting to come into my awareness.

After the hospital, I kept thinking about how my parents didn't ever seem to be together in my memory. What was going on with them, between them, to treat me as they did? Did either of them know what the other had been doing? For that matter, what was going on with my siblings? Especially the ones who were ten, twelve, fifteen, and seventeen years older than me. What did they know?

"Is it weird that I have no memory of my parents together—in any way? I can't recall them being together. In my life at all. I can't picture them in the same room ever. No mental images of them at the same meal table. I have no memories of them abusing me together. And— why were my fantasies only about a father? Never a fantasy mother?"

I would spend many sessions searching inside for an answer. There was a dynamic that caused the little girls, including little Sally, to be glued to my mother. Some were afraid to lose her or be away from her; some terrified of being in her presence. But all of them were terrified of my father and hated him.

It had also become clear to me, over the course of my work with Dr. Siegel, that the memories of sexual abuse from my mom were all in the DC house. Her physical abuse continued in Chapel Hill—the whippings and beatings, the screaming, her drunkenness. But not the sexual abuse. With my father, my memories of sexual abuse were in both DC and Chapel Hill. But he'd stopped coming to my room in Chapel Hill at some point. Why?

"Dr. Siegel, why did they stop at different times? What happened? Why did any of it stop? And why wasn't I able to think of a single word about my relationship with my mother, while I felt so much terror about my dad in those early sessions with you?"

I really wanted to make sense of all these questions. At a certain point, I came to realize that there was a limit to making sense—and that limit lay with my parents' actions. That I hadn't been able to make sense of their actions—that I felt *fear without solution*, as Dr. Siegel had explained— was at the heart of why I had developed MPD. The MPD, really, was how I *had* made sense of it, to the extent I could have. I *had* to fragment and have states that could be ready for all of it. All in all, in my mind, MPD was looking less and less like a disorder, more and more like a life preserver—the very life preserver that Dr. Siegel had first told me it was. A brilliant adaptation. A life-saving response to unspeakably disturbed, cruel, and horrific abuse within an incestuous family.

Horrific, abusive, cruel family disorder.

It didn't make any sense. MPD was the only way *to* make sense of it.

Still, I struggled with this for some time—looking for answers I probably would never get. What must it have been like for all of them? I couldn't answer that question on my own, especially with no one willing to offer even the slightest bit of insight, much less validation.

With time, things would surface that gave me some answers—or, if not answers, information. Some of my family's secrets and denials would surface. But that wouldn't be for years.

ONE MORNING IN THE SUMMER OF 1994, I had an early appointment with Dr. Siegel. When I first walked in, he told me he had some news to report. There was a change taking place in the clinical view of MPD.

"Officially now, Sally, MPD will be known and diagnosed as Dissociative Identity Disorder, or DID."

The salient difference was that with MPD, "fragmentation" was seen as the development of distinct personalities. DID, on the other hand, was characterized by the emergence not of personalities, but states of mind.

To some, this might've seemed a rather subtle difference. But DID, as a concept, did resonate with me more than MPD. As much as I could see it as adaptive, MPD had also felt like an unhealthy deficit as the result of early abuse—like a shattering of self. DID felt truer to the reality I'd come to discover—that fragmentation was really a healthy response to the unhealthiest circumstances for a child. My own experience always felt like one of states, not personalities, and that is how Dr. Siegel had treated me from the start. As he described it to me,

"We all have many different states of mind—when we're driving, as opposed to teaching a class, or playing tennis, as opposed to shopping at the grocery store. For MPD—or now, DID—the distinction is there are memory barriers between states of mind. When I'm at the grocery store, for instance, I remember I just came from a tennis match. For DID patients, there is no such continuity of memory, which is what makes the operation of the states problematic—what was once highly adaptive becomes maladaptive. Once continuity of memory is established, Sally—as you are beginning to experience—integration and recovery is possible."

It was all *making sense* to me, and I welcomed the change. It felt more reflective of all I was experiencing. *My brilliant, adaptive, protective states of mind.*

WITH THE NEW PERSPECTIVE OF DID, Dr. Siegel and I were talking about the changes in me we were both noticing. Lately, when I would look inside for answers, as I'd been doing for so long, I was coming up blank. It felt strange.

"Do you think the states have all left, Dr. Siegel?"

"What do you think?"

"You know what I think?"

"Tell me."

"I think they're all there...but they aren't so separate, since the hospital. And now they want me to find some of these answers for myself. Not in a mean or withholding way, but as you describe integration. They're linked and working together—joining forces to know it all and make sense of it all. Does that make sense?"

"I think it makes a lot of sense, Sally."

Dr. Siegel had talked to me about integration over the years, but I'd never been sure what it would feel like. As he explained, integration was a state of mental well-being, and emotional regulation. It wasn't just for DID patients. For him, integration was the hallmark of emotional well-being for everyone...individuals, families, couples, organizations, even governments. It was also the goal of therapy—the linkage of differentiated elements, like parts or states, which allowed people to experience better physical health, less burnout, more intentional strength, and greater relational empathy. And now, I was beginning to not just understand it—I was feeling it. Feeling the connection of my states, with their distinct ways of processing information, into a functional whole. A whole, functional, integrated me.

"Do I lose the different states?" I asked him now.

"I think what happens is you maintain what the states of mind know..."

"How they saved me?"

"Yes. And as they become linked, the memory barriers dissolve, so there's no more separation."

I loved the metaphor he used to explain this process. "Do you remember when Sam stopped crawling and started walking?"

"Yes! What a great day that was—on Paul's birthday, just about two months after we got home from Romania. Right before we met you at UCLA."

"Beautiful. When he started walking, what happened to the crawling Sam? Was he lost, forgotten?"

"No," I said. "I see. Integration."

"That's right—all the states will share the same memories. It might help to think of your different states as verbs, Sally, not nouns. You aren't separate people, as in the old MPD misunderstanding—you're one person, and the states are verbs that acted to protect you, as a person, from a family that didn't protect you."

Another metaphor occurred to me. "Like sentries, guarding my core happiness?"

"Beautifully said."

As I left his office, I was feeling—not chaos, or rigidity; I was feeling that things were changing. That feeling of happiness was very much in my awareness. Happiness as a verb. A capacity; the experience of an integrated state of mind.

ON THANKSGIVING DAY, 1994, Paul, Sam, and I had been with friends for the holiday dinner. Not long after we got home, the phone rang. I answered. At first I didn't recognize the voice—it was my brother-in-law, whom I hadn't spoken to since before the it's-not-denial-if-it-never-happened call with his wife, my oldest sister.

"Sally?"

"Yes?"

He told me who it was.

"I'm calling to let you know that your father has passed away."

"Thanks for letting me know," I said, and hung up. It was the strangest feeling—kind of like that old straddling between two worlds. But I didn't disappear—I didn't dissociate—I was fully present to what I'd just heard. I just wasn't sure quite what it meant to me.

Paul was right there. "Who was that?"

For the very briefest moment, I felt the possibility of a tear. A single tear. And then, before it even came close to leaving my tear duct, it disappeared.

"It was my brother-in-law. My dad died."

"Oh. You okay, Sal?"

I took a minute—checked inside.

"Yes, yes. I am. I'm okay."

Paul looked back at me with a question on his face.

"Really, Paul—I'm okay." I really didn't have any more to say about it. I was done.

Paul came over and hugged me. I was relieved. He was too.

LATER, IN DR. SIEGEL'S OFFICE, I told him about what had happened, and about the tear.

"Can you tell me how you're feeling?"

"Relief. I'm feeling relieved."

The world just felt a little safer, with him no longer in it.

DR. SIEGEL AND I got to talking more about memory—memory and my happiness. It really bothered me that, apart from being at the swimming pool in the summer, and despite Peggy's fantasy about the tree and the loving father who might save me, I couldn't come up with any actual happy memories from childhood—yet I had a sense of happiness at my core. How could that have been? Weren't there any other actually good, happy memories in there, somewhere?

At Dr. Siegel's suggestion, I scrolled through my memory—holidays? Christmas? Easter? Halloween? I had no memories—or no good memories—of any holiday.

He asked me, "What were your birthdays like?"

That question jogged a memory. It felt like something I had forgotten but then remembered—so maybe I hadn't ever really forgotten it? "Well, there was the time my oldest sister took me on my fifth birthday to see Disney's *Sleeping Beauty*. It was the first time I'd been to the movies. I loved the three magic fairies and how they took care of the baby princess. How they could disappear at will with their magic wands when they needed to for safety.

"Other than that, I don't think my birthdays were ever much fun."

Looking inside, it felt like Jennifer, Sarah, Allison, Jessica, and even Peggy let me know that in my family, there wasn't much happiness or fun.

"I wonder if there were happy moments for anyone in that family, ever, Dr. Siegel."

Also, there seemed to be a collective awareness that no one in that house—except for my oldest sister, maybe—was happy I was born.

The one possible exception: I did unearth this vague memory of when we still lived in DC—so, before I was eight—and my oldest brother was coming over. I don't know if it was for Christmas, my birthday, or even a special occasion. I remember he brought me a present.

"That's the first time I have any memory of meeting him."

"He didn't live at your house?"

"I don't ever remember him there."

I had no memory of him before this time, and I'm not sure I understood his relationship to me. He was much older than me—seventeen years older.

As much as I was searching for information about this visit from my brother, I was more and more and more aware of how this information was coming to me. It was from my memory. It was vague and a little fuzzy—but I was remembering it without a state's help.

"What I remember, from much later in my life—I think my oldest sister told me—is that when I was born, my father and brother had a big fight. My father kicked him out, and I think this visit was the first time he'd been back."

"Do you know why he got kicked out?"

"No, I don't know why. He'd joined the Army or Air Force and was getting ready to go overseas, I think, when he came to visit. He brought me stationery with my name on it. And then I didn't see him again until we moved to Chapel Hill," I said. "He came for a short visit. He was married by then and had two children. I was probably ten."

I was looking deeper and deeper, and another memory kind of peeked out—took me a little by surprise.

"It was in DC, I was little."

"How little?"

"Four or five. I think my mom would take me to see him at the store he worked in. It was a shoe store, I think."

I was sitting there with my eyes closed...remembering.

"I think my mom was taking me and I had to keep it secret. I don't think she wanted my dad to know."

"Do you know why she wouldn't want him to know?"

"Not really."

I suddenly remembered something else about that brother. I think I was eleven or twelve and my parents, my two-years-older sister, and I had driven from our home in Chapel Hill to Los Angeles to visit him and his family. And then—"I think I've found a happy memory," I said, because I had. "We went to Disneyland!"

I was so happy to have remembered this. Dr. Siegel looked almost as excited as I did.

"I still don't seem to have any memories about being together with any family members there. But I remember how I felt when I was there. I have a real sense that Disneyland was everything I wanted it to be."

"Explain a little more about that, if you can."

I closed my eyes. I could picture myself there. I could picture Main Street. The characters. Sleeping Beauty's Castle. And I could remember, too, how excited I'd been before we went, in anticipation of finally getting to see it. "I was counting the days until we got there."

"To California? To see your brother and his family?"

"No. I barely remember seeing them. I was counting the minutes to get to Disneyland."

The happiest place on earth.

I sat back, eyes closed, and looked inside for a memory of me at Disneyland that included even one member of my family.

"Nothing, Dr. Siegel. Not one memory coming about them there with me. I know they were there with me, but I don't remember that."

I was in a little bit of a daze. I wasn't crying. I was more in...I was kind of blank.

"What are you thinking about, Sally?"

"Just how empty that family was."

"Yes."

"No sense of connection, or joy, or...happiness with them. Nothing—only feelings of fear, emptiness, terror and...disgust...about that family. My family."

Just sat for a minute. Eyes closed. And then I opened them and said what then occurred to me: "I think it's a happy memory because I don't remember them."

Thank you, Peggy, Jennifer, Sarah. Thank you all for preserving what was good.

Dr. Siegel was there with me, understanding this very fresh awareness.

"I must've been so lonely."

"Yes."

"I think the states kept me company."

I was remembering being happy within myself—with their help. They were the guardians.

It was at that point that I started to think that perhaps the absence of my family members from my happiest memories wasn't an aberration. Maybe it reflected the way that the sentries of my DID wouldn't allow the poison of that toxic, abusive family to seep into the deepest part of me. With their help, I was happy in my core. I was happy to remember about Disneyland.

THAT WEEKEND, I took Sam to Disneyland.

We flew out of Wendy Darling's nursery window.

Got "It's a Small World After All" looping in our ears.

Sam saw Mickey walking down Main Street and ran toward him, and Mickey caught him in a huge embrace.

And I was happy to simply stand in the center of Sleeping Beauty's Castle.

This is the stuff of happy childhoods.

I bought a videotape of *Sleeping Beauty* to see the fairies.

Sam said the birthday cake the fairies made for the princess looked a lot like the birthday cakes I made him.

He was right.

WITH ALL THE NEW INFORMATION AND INSIGHT, therapy had begun to feel lighter. Communication within, even as I jumped around in time and place, had taken on a new sense of ease; I wasn't getting so lost.

As Dr. Siegel and I were speaking more about that trip with my family, I remembered something else. It took me a little while to make sense of it.

"Can you tell me what you're remembering, Sally?"

"I am remembering, Dr. Siegel, that the sexual and physical abuse stopped after that trip."

"Why do you think that was, Sally?"

I closed my eyes—not so much to search, but simply to ask for the answer. This was one of the big differences in therapy now, in my state of increased integration—I could just ask, and answers would often enter my awareness.

"Can you tell me what you're remembering?"

"Yes." It was a clear memory—again, almost as if I had never forgotten—kind of like a revelation.

"On that trip, Dr. Siegel, I faked starting my period."

I had cut my finger, put blood on my underwear, and told my mother. I don't know if I knew that would stop him, or if that was even what motivated me. But I remember really wanting to start my period, so I faked it. And it worked.

"I don't know if that's *why* he stopped, Dr. Siegel, but my father never hurt me sexually again."

I wouldn't actually start my period until I was in eighth grade at age fourteen.

"I have a strong sense, Dr. Siegel, that I was still very afraid of him after that, but I don't have much memory of being around him. Almost like I had some protection."

"Protection?"

"I don't know exactly—I can remember that once we moved to Galveston when I was fifteen and in high school—and most of my friends there could drive, I was able to be away from home more. Somehow I was able to avoid him."

"Do you know how that worked?"

Suddenly, but gently, a new state became known to me.

The Invisible state.

The Invisible state did not have much of a voice.

"I think she may have been born when I was really little, out of this stupid game my family played where they would pretend not to be able to see me even when I was right in front of them."

I hated that game.

Invisible could speak softly, but mostly she just let me know her thoughts. When I was so little, Invisible helped me disappear into my tree when I heard the steps getting closer. When I was older, she helped me just by figuring out how I could keep out of his way as much as possible.

Another revelation. "You know what, Dr. Siegel?"

"What, Sally?"

"When Paul and I got married, most of my family came, and I have almost no memory of it. When we got our pictures back, there were hardly any of me."

"What do you think of that?"

"I kind of remember feeling invisible—really—like I could see everyone, but no one could see me."

Protection.

We both just kind of sat there, quiet, for a few moments, as though we were admiring the power and creativity of my child's mind.

"Your mind really took care of you, Sally."

After a while, Sarah had something to add—it was her hatred that helped me keep them at a distance, too. The combo of Sarah and Invisible are what allowed me to never need my family and to stay away from home as much as possible, from our time in Galveston onward.

I also think it's possible that neither of my parents was interested in sex or violence that involved any kind of resistance. And as I entered adolescence, resistance was my primary drive.

Thank you, Sarah.

Dr. Siegel talked a little about what happens to the brain—not just the DID brain, but all brains—in adolescence. How the brain is naturally moving you away from family—how it's time to separate from them, to figure out how to make it on your own. Staying away from home as a teenager was what made high school in Galveston ultimately good for me.

"Can you tell me more about what life was like then?" Dr. Siegel asked.

"Well, in high school, I was still afraid and really cautious—but not as afraid as when I was younger."

"Do you know why that was?"

I paused to allow an answer to come to me.

"In Chapel Hill, even once the sexual abuse stopped after that trip, going through puberty made me feel so exposed and vulnerable. I was so aware, Dr. Siegel, of the changes in my body. Embarrassed to have a body. I hated my body. It humiliated me. All the time. But by the time I got to Galveston to start tenth grade, with the reality and threat of the sexual abuse gone..."

I had to think about this for a moment...

"It wasn't so dangerous to have a body."

Wow.

"What an awareness, Sally." Dr. Siegel and I both were kind of smiling at the idea of my body no longer being a threat to me.

"My memories in Galveston are about life outside the house. I had a good, solid group of friends. We did everything together. My best friends all had boyfriends, and I loved being with them. We all hung out together. I felt like I belonged."

We were sitting there, talking. I was more in the chair these days than on the couch. And as we talked, I had this gentle flash of a memory. I closed my eyes, and Dr. Siegel asked me what was going on.

"Oh my."

"What, Sally?"

"I'm remembering something I want to share with you."

More and more, memories were coming to me this way, in spontaneous but welcome waves. This was a good one.

It was my junior year of high school. Galveston. On a Saturday night, one of my best friends, who had a car, picked me up. And instead of going to one of our usual hangouts with friends, she wanted to go to her new boyfriend's house. I didn't really want to go. His family had only just moved there, and his father worked with my father. But it was her car, her boyfriend. I was just along for the ride.

Her boyfriend had lots of brothers and sisters. After just a little time there, I found his parents to be the nicest parents I'd ever met. Hanging out at their house felt good. So, I started to hang out there with them often. His dad, in particular, had been so nice. He always made a point to ask me how school was. Once I let him know I was worried about a test I had taken, and the next time he saw me he asked,

"Sally, how'd you do on that test?"

He'd remembered.

It warmed my heart to remember it now.

One night we were over there, and I noticed their daughter, who was just fourteen, wasn't home. She had a reputation for being wild, and I wondered where she was. At some point the phone rang and I could tell from her dad's conversation it was the police. She had been picked up with an older boy, in a van, smoking pot and making out. The police, who knew the dad, were calling to say they'd be happy to bring her home, but also fine to throw her in the slammer if he wanted to teach her a lesson.

"I would so appreciate it if you would bring her home, officer."

I immediately wanted to leave. I knew what was about to happen. I didn't want to be there for that, and I begged my friend to leave. She didn't want to. Her boyfriend said it was fine to stay. I was a nervous wreck. When the doorbell rang, the dad went to open it. I heard him thank the officers. She walked in and he came in behind her.

I was standing there with my heart in my throat—terrified for what was to come.

He shut the door behind him...and then...he hugged her.

He hugged her.

"Dr. Siegel—he hugged her!"

"What was that like for you, Sally?"

"I never knew that was an option."

"What a memory, Sally."

"Yes. You know, I would've been killed if that had been my father."

Quiet tears kind of trickled down my face.

"Tell me about those tears."

"He was so nice to me."

"It sounds like he offered you a new mental model of what family could mean. He hugged her. You never knew that was an option. How did that impact you—seeing a new way?"

"It took a while to sink in—but yes, it gave me hope that things could be different. Hope that I could be different."

That life could be different.

"You know what I'm remembering right now?"

"Tell me."

"I have this vision of me. I'm with the boyfriend I told you about in the padded room. We'd been to the movies, and he was dropping me off at my house."

I started to really cry.

"What's happening, Sally?"

"I'm just standing there. Looking at the front door."

It was such a vivid memory. I could feel it.

"I just can't go in. I hate it in there."

By then, I was old enough to realize I could avoid them sometimes. But I was still only sixteen. I couldn't just disappear. I still had to survive in there.

"Dr. Siegel."

"Yes, Sally. I'm right here."

"It was an awful place to live."

"I know it was."

"Dr. Siegel."

"What, Sally?"

"Could we do some guided imagery? Do we have time?"

"Certainly. What are you wanting?"

"It feels like I need to look at more inside." I wasn't sure why; I just felt a need. I was learning to trust those feelings. "Can we try?"

"Yes, we can."

I got comfortable on the couch. No blanket now; just a pillow under my head and one in my lap.

"Just take some breaths now, Sally."

Breathing in...out...intentional...

In our guided imagery sessions, Dr. Siegel would take me to a safe place of my choosing. It was most often a place alongside a river where Paul and I had been with friends. It had a special meaning to me and felt so deeply connected and safe. Life was good there.

"Imagine," said Dr. Siegel, leading me through the imagery exercise as he always did, "there is a white light that surrounds you. Nothing bad can happen to you here. You can be relaxed and just allow whatever arises to come into your awareness."

I was completely relaxed. Breathing in and breathing out. Being curious and open to whatever might come. It felt like I was floating. I could see myself floating through my life. I remembered all the boys in high school I had crushes on and how I could never allow myself physical and sexual closeness. Or if I did have sex, and even enjoy it, as happened once in high school and a couple of times in college, I could never look at the guy again and would just pretend it didn't happen. I have no idea what any of them thought of me. It was crazy. I could see my friends, too, and how they were with their families, and how I loved being at other people's houses—never at mine. I could see how there was happiness just under my surface and how I had to keep it close so as not to lose it. I could never show it at home. It was not safe to be happy at home. I could see how I had found ways to keep my family away from me. And how even when they were the most intrusive, I had ways to not know it.

"I think I'm going to have to hold my breath for a minute, Dr. Siegel."

"Okay—can I help?"

I was crying. Quiet tears. I knew something was coming. I knew I needed his help.

"Dr. Siegel."

"Yes, Sally."

"I'm afraid to ask you something."

"You can ask me anything, Sally."

"Could you hold my hand for a minute?"

He moved his chair closer to me on the couch and took my hand.

Suddenly I felt as if I was in the ocean. I was completely submerged and being tossed all over. I couldn't breathe. It felt dangerous. I could feel the parts of my body that had been so hurt as a little girl. I could feel it all. I was being scraped on the bottom of the ocean. Hurting. Feeling like I had to fight for my life. Feeling all the longing of things lost. The wishes for connection. The nights of absolute fear. The pure feelings of terror and anger and hatred and wishes for something better. I could feel Dr. Siegel holding my hand. Suddenly I could breathe. And I was on the sandy bottom of the ocean. It was calm. I was calm. I was breathing. I could feel, all at once, a warm, soothing stream of water, and then a cool, refreshing one. Suddenly I could see all the way up to the surface of the ocean. The waves that had been tossing me around, devouring me, trying to drown me, were now calm. The water looked more like a lake now. I let go of Dr. Siegel's hand and swam to the surface. I took a big giant breath. I was okay.

It was as if all my differentiated states were collectively showing me everything they knew. How they'd worked so hard to save me. And I could see it. I could know it. And even though it was still hard, it was all making sense, and that made all the difference.

"I can know it, Dr. Siegel. I can know it."

"I know you can, Sally."

"What are you thinking, Dr. Siegel?"

He paused, closed his eyes. Sighed. Opened his eyes to look at me.

"What I think so often in the work you're doing, Sally. That you're so very brave. That you've endured so much and you're working so hard at understanding. I think you're amazing, Sally. I have great admiration for you."

We both just sat there. It was a lot to take in. And I knew that with his support, I could be okay with all that happened.

I KEPT FEELING THAT EASE of internal communication, growing easier all the time. It was the experience of integration, as the differentiated states of my mind were being honored and linking together as I was learning to still my internal waters to calm. I could feel it, just as Dr. Siegel had described it earlier. My memory was working in a new way. It felt natural. Connected. Energized. *Free.*

I was more and more curious to know why my parents had been so cruel to me. I believe now that some of my siblings had been abused as well. I had come to understand that my father was, plain and simple, a brutal and sadistic man. I had clear memories of him being drunk. He would kick and beat our dog and whip his children with a belt in a ritualistic way—he enjoyed it. I strongly suspect my mother had DID. Of course I can't say for certain, but my memories of her are that she had many different ways of being with me. Sometimes caring, sometimes needing care, and then horribly abusive in all ways, including sexually. They were both monsters. I hated them both. But sometimes, I felt sad and sorry for my mother. It was complicated for me.

But there was something about me that my father particularly hated. Why? And no one had been especially happy I'd been born. At one point I thought maybe I wasn't my mother's baby. Could I have been my oldest sister's? Was that why she'd seemed to care about me in ways that no one else had? But that meant she would've been eleven when I was conceived. Seemed unlikely. I ruled that possibility out.

In one session, I was remembering about how my oldest brother, whom I'd last seen when I was eleven, during that trip to Disneyland, had moved to Galveston after his divorce and lived with us.

"What was it like, Sally, having him live there?"

"I was always a little uncomfortable around him. I'm not sure why. Just my normal feelings around that family, I guess."

"Can you describe what you mean by 'normal'?"

"Well—you know. A little creepy. Had to be vigilant. There were a couple times I'm remembering now when I felt like he was getting a little too close."

"Close in what way?"

I had to think for a minute. Closing my eyes. Getting that creepy feeling. A little twitchy.

"I think he may have made a sexual move at one point."

Going a little deeper looking...curious...open.

"Yeah. I think that he may have...um...kind of reached to kiss me... and I just retreated immediately."

I didn't freeze.

Thank you, Jessica. I'm sorry you had to deal with that on top of everything else.

I opened my eyes. Then remembered something more.

"It was tricky with him, though."

"Tricky how?"

"I hated my sister, who was two years older. If I was in tenth grade then, she was in twelfth. She was just awful. Kind of creepy. A fucking tattletale. Terrible to deal with. I just never liked her. Ever."

Oh god.

"She made life miserable at times."

"How?"

"She just was mean and intrusive."

"In what way intrusive, Sally?"

"Nothing sexual. With me. I mean, maybe when we were little. But not by high school. She was no threat. I just didn't like her."

Now, I can see how troubled she must've been, to behave as she'd behaved. But then, I had no insight into our family. So, I just stayed as clear of her as best I could.

"Maybe why I hated her so much was because in her I could see how fucked up that family was."

A constant reminder.

Ick.

"But with my brother living there for a while, well—he was kind of a buffer between us. He could be fun. And I don't think he liked her either. She was no fun. He smoked and drank and would drive me around. Give me rides. I kind of tolerated him."

"Were you afraid of him?"

"No—he was a little creepy, but not dangerous. I mean, he wasn't so much creepy really, even. Just made me uncomfortable when he'd try to get too close."

I closed my eyes and began to remember some other things about him.

"He came to Galveston because he needed a job, and he went to work for my father. There was no relationship between them that I recall. Again, no memory at all of them together. He and mom were close...but they fought a lot. I mean screaming matches."

"Do you know what they fought about?"

I had to think about it for a minute.

"About his ex-wife. Mom hated her. And his kids. He left his kids in California. I don't think they ever came to visit him in Galveston. Maybe once."

Again, closing my eyes. Remembering things about that time. It must've been when I was sixteen and lasted a couple of years. I don't remember him being in the house much when I was a senior. I think by then he'd moved to his own place. Then suddenly I was thinking how he'd been kicked out of the house around the same time I was born. And how my mom would sneak me to see him. How it was like a secret outing she and I would take. Our little secret. She'd be really nice then. And he'd brought me that present. He might've brought others presents too, but the only one I could remember was the one he'd brought me.

"You know, Dr. Siegel, everyone always said how much his daughter and I looked alike."

"What are you thinking, Sally?"

I took a moment to breathe. Not because I felt dizzy or lost—quite the opposite. It felt like I may have figured something out, and that as crazy as it sounded—made sense.

"You know what, Dr. Siegel?"

"Tell me."

"I wonder if my big brother might be my father."

It felt like we both may have simultaneously gasped.

We talked about it over a few sessions. Just putting pieces of the puzzle together. Fact-checking as well as I could. More and more, it seemed to make sense.

Making sense of the nonsensical.

Again.

At the end of the session I said to Dr. Siegel,

"I'm going to call and ask him."

IT TOOK A COUPLE OF DAYS for me to track down a number for him. He lived kind of an unstable life. Then I found an old number for him—it worked!

I called him.

He answered.

I said hello. He said howdy back.

I got right to the point.

"Hey, I'm wondering if you think it's possible that Mom and Dad were abusive to me? Sexually abusive?"

He took a little time to answer.

"Yes, I do believe that's absolutely a possibility."

"Do you remember them being abusive to me? Were they abusive to you?"

Suddenly realizing I was at the source of so much family history, I had so many questions to ask him, hope, hope, hoping for answers, wishing for some truth.

He told me that he knew the family to have a history of abusive and incestuous behavior. But he avoided giving any direct answers about himself or offering any specifics about me. All he said was,

"If you remember it happening, trust yourself, Sally."

He told me about our aunts, whom everyone, including themselves, had referred to as "old maids," and said they were lovers. They'd lived together for most of their adult lives. And he remembered, as a little kid, visiting them one summer and walking in on them having sex.

A little truth felt good.

He was the first one to ever confirm anything I knew.

Then I called him by name and just blurted it out,

"Is it possible you're my father?"

After a moment's hesitation, he finally answered,

"Well, I'll tell you what I know for sure—that..."

...and he said my mother's full name here...

"...is your mother."

What?

"What does that mean?"

"It means what it means. I gotta go."

And he hung up.

I would never see him again.

"What do you think about that, Sally?"

"What do I think, or feel?"

"Both...either."

"What does it feel like to think that it's a possibility that I'm...oh my god...the child of my mother and my...fuck...my brother?"

It was the first time I had said it out loud.

"Yes."

I kind of laughed, very quietly...inwardly.

"You know, like so many other things, Dr. Siegel—so counterintuitive—it feels lucky just to know that the fucking sadistic father is not... my father."

Fuck him.

I fucking hate him.

I'm so glad he's dead.

"I mean really, Dr. Siegel—when the good news is that your brother and mother are your parents...well..."

"Well what?"

"It speaks for itself."

"What does it feel like for him to have validated your questions about family abuse?"

"Good. It's good to have some validation of a sort."

"The truth is your friend."

Yes, it is.

"You know, at first, I was going to say, 'but the truth hurts'...but I don't think that's true any longer."

"What do you mean?"

"The truth is just the truth."

"And you've been seeking the truth for a long time now, Sally."

Yes. I have.

Thank you, Dr. Siegel. Thank you for guiding me.

The truth is setting me free.

PART 4

BY THE SUMMER OF 1997, after six years of therapy with Dr. Siegel, the intensity of our sessions had eased. Our focus was now on the present—on me being the mom of an eight-year-old Sam, who was growing more independent.

As the states communicated directly within me, DID was no longer the center of our work. I could talk to Dr. Siegel about anything without feelings of shame, fear, or doubt. We did at times reflect on the painful work we had done, and he would check in with me occasionally for safety purposes. But I was starting to feel good about myself and about life. And as we talked about what the work we'd done in therapy meant to me, I was exploring the idea of going back to school to earn a master's degree in clinical psychology. Dr. Siegel was supportive of the idea. I was checking out my options.

One day in June I got a call—this time from a niece I hadn't had much contact with—to tell me my mother had died. I was at home when I got the call. Unlike with the news that the man I'd thought was my father had died, I didn't experience even the promise of a tear at the news of my mother's death. I breathed a little easier knowing she was off the planet.

Dr. Siegel and I didn't spend much time on it. My grieving wouldn't have been for her, but for the loss of my childhood, and I was done with that now. But there was one thing I wanted to do.

"I'd like to check in with the states," I told him. "Make sure they all know. And see if they have anything they might want your help with."

"Great idea. How shall we start?"

Even six months ago I would've asked for some grounding focus or guided imagery. This time I didn't need to go so deep for a check-in. I knew the states' thoughts. I was more and more aware of the feeling of integration.

Their thoughts about her death filled my awareness. They were my thoughts.

Jennifer knew and was pleased for me to finally have some relief from the horrors of that family. She felt pride in getting me to Dr. Siegel.

She believed her work was done. She felt relief the mother was dead. Relieved to no longer worry about that.

Allison too was glad. She'd been instrumental in freeing me from the grip of the sexual abuse—the death came as good news.

Sarah was very glad. *Ding-dong, the wicked witch is dead.* She had held the hate and anger to keep me safe. I thanked her and told her she could let it all go. Both parents were dead. She could feel safe.

Jessica was happy. I thanked her for propelling me out of that family model with so much spunk and vigor. *Fuck them.* I was sorry about the boyfriends, and I let her know she'd helped me figure things out; I was no longer afraid of sex. That made her happy.

Little Sally was still little and sad that the mother was dead. She was grieving. I was able to help her by mothering her as I did Sam. Dr. Siegel let her know I was a good mom; I'd mothered myself, too. And so Little Sally was sad, but safe.

No-Body was happy for all she'd contributed. And she was ready to join my body. I welcomed her.

The angry parts remembered their anger and were relieved she was gone.

The part that hated the body felt better knowing she was gone.

The Just Blank state believed she'd already stopped being Blank— and was feeling feelings. As Dr. Siegel had told me, one of his goals for our therapy had been for all the states to have ever-widening windows of tolerance. Here, it was clear that goal had been achieved.

Peggy remained happy.

The only states I couldn't get a read on were the little girls. But Dr. Siegel and I wanted to honor their privacy, something they had never had, inviting them to let us know how they felt when they were ready.

I felt sure they would let us know.

NOT LONG AFTER MY MOTHER'S DEATH, I saw a news story about a mom who'd jumped off a bridge, taking her small children with her. It startled me. I was feeling uncomfortable in my own skin, thinking about it.

I told Dr. Siegel about it.

"I have this feeling that…I mean…not that…not that I want to kill myself—and certainly not to put Sam in any danger. But…"

"But what, Sally?"

"My first thought was, 'How could any mother do that?'—but then I thought, 'Of course she took them with her.'"

"Tell me what you mean, please."

"I had this overwhelming feeling that she would have to keep her children with her. How could she leave them behind?"

I wasn't crying, but I was really upset. He could see how upset I was. I just couldn't understand why this story was having such an impact on me. I didn't feel safe—that was alarming to Dr. Siegel. It was alarming to me, too.

"Sally, I think we need to do this work in the hospital." Again, something scary was happening and we needed to figure it out. Safety first.

He made the arrangements. This time, no confusion. No hesitation. No sharps. No cigarettes.

I checked in to the same unit. Different staff, and patients. Different issues to explore than the Jessica hospital stay, but certainly the same needs for safety.

The first night was not as hard as the time before, but I was scared. Thinking I'd come so far. Only to experience—what? A setback? Breakdown? Was I a cautionary tale?

I checked in on a Sunday and would see Dr. Siegel in the morning. Once settled in, I heard the staff was taking the girls to the athletic field for a walk. I felt anxious. Some fresh air sounded good—I asked to join them.

The nurse said he needed to check with Dr. Siegel first.

I was in my room when the nurse came in to tell me Dr. Siegel said it was fine, but he wanted me to search inside to make sure I'd be safe, and that there was no risk of me running away. It startled me a little—*flight risk?*—but I understood.

I asked the nurse to give me a little time to check inside.

I closed my eyes. Deep dive. I had thought things were calmer than they were. Inside, it was eerily quiet. I wasn't sure why, but I remembered telling Dr. Siegel once about being in the orphanage in Romania, and how strangely quiet it could be. No sounds of babies. He had told me that when babies cry and repeatedly no one responds, they will stop crying—stop asking for help. I wasn't sure what was going on, but instinct told me there was something happening to me, inside, now. And I needed to pay attention to it. So, I let the nurse know I would skip the walk. I was erring on the side of safety.

Flight risk.

Once Dr. Siegel arrived in the morning, we got to work.

No padded room this time. Just a room.

Over the next two days, we discovered that some of the little girls from the green blanket were feeling deeply alone, abandoned, and so, so sad. The news of the death of my mother had not been easy for them.

No wonder I couldn't find them when I checked.

They were despondent.

When they'd heard about my mother's death, they hadn't understood why she'd left without them. And then, hearing about the mother who'd taken her children with her sent them spiraling into a deep sadness and feelings of abandonment. The states that had been relieved, even joyful that the mother was gone were furious. The little girls' reaction upset them—they were wishing she *had* taken them with her.

Mean-girl mean.

Dr. Siegel got us all communicating.

Validating emotions.

For all states.

It's okay to be sad.

It's okay to be mad.

Mad and sad.

Two opposite emotions at once.

Words of comfort for all.

And for me: "This isn't a setback, Sally—more of a turning point. It's all progress."

And again, he let it be known that there was a mother available to all, including the little girls. Not their mother—she was gone. But I was a mother now, and I cared about them just as I did for Sam.

It was healing for them.

Healing for me.

At the end of the final session before going home—after only three days—I had a question I wanted to ask Dr. Siegel. "Why do you think I've been able to be a good mom, after growing up in that family?"

I was expecting him to ask me why *I* thought I had turned out to be a good mom.

He surprised me.

"You know what I think, Sally?"

"What, Dr. Siegel?"

"I think you've become the mother you always wished you could've had."

I think he was right.

I'd become a mother not just for Sam, but for me—all of me. The kind of parent I'd dreamed of.

That made Peggy happy.

Me too.

Breakthrough.

"DO YOU REMEMBER TELLING ME, DR. SIEGEL, I would notice the feeling of being whole one day?"

"I do remember telling you that, Sally."

"I think it's happening."

"Can you describe it to me?" He genuinely seemed pleased.

"You know how you talk about that 'bring it on' feeling?"

"Yes! The stance that invites anything from anywhere to enter awareness without moving out of your window of tolerance?"

I smiled. "Yes! That's how I'm feeling now. I have a clarity of vision. I know I had a childhood full of pain, but don't feel it. I feel grounded in the here and now, and I'm connecting to a sense of what can happen in the future.

Making sense...integration...no memory barriers...

"Does that mean I've recovered from DID?

"A big yes, Sally. That sounds like recovery to me."

What a moment. It was incredible to sit there with Dr. Siegel, knowing all we had accomplished. Sitting in the quiet, knowing all we had done, I couldn't describe how grateful I was—but I did feel it. I think he felt it too.

THE ONLY CHALLENGES REMAINING were occasional intrusive thoughts. I thought of them as rogue memories. They weren't new; I recognized them immediately, where they came from. They weren't disturbing, not in the way they'd once been, but they could still throw me off course. I didn't like it. What had been adaptive, doorways into knowledge I'd needed to make sense of, was now simply maladaptive. Disruptive.

One morning, Dr. Siegel let me know he was back from a training with Dr. Francine Shapiro at UC Berkeley, where he'd learned about her new trauma therapy, EMDR. He was enthusiastic about it and wondered if I'd like to try it.

"I think it might be helpful with the lingering intrusive memories, Sally."

"How does it work?"

He explained that Dr. Shapiro had found great success with trauma patients using rapid-eye movements that she believed replicated REM sleep, which typically promoted the processing of unresolved—and traumatic—memories. EMDR proved remarkably helpful for me. So much so that while I don't recall exactly what the intrusive thoughts we worked on were, I clearly remember the process. First, I'd describe an intrusive memory—where I noticed it in my body and what emotions came with it, and any images that came to mind. Was there a negative thought about myself it brought up? What positive thought would I like to have instead?

Then, we'd sit across from each other, my eyes open. Dr. Siegel would move his first two fingers rapidly in front of me as I tracked them back and forth with my eyes, keeping my head still. What I remember most was that immediately tears would come gushing...and eventually, I would almost always end up laughing—out loud. As best as I recall, after every single session, the intrusive thoughts and memories we'd been working with disappeared. Forever.

By the time I was being trained in EMDR as a clinician, some years later, it had been determined that the mechanism at work in EMDR is bilateral stimulation, which could also be achieved using right/left taps or alternating sound tones, with the same remarkable results of desensitizing distressing memories, thus reducing their emotional intensity.

LIFE WAS GETTING EASIER. I'd come such a long way in what was seven years now. Dr. Siegel and I weren't meeting as often; the feelings of safety and clarity, of having made sense of my story, kept growing stronger. One day in his office, I wanted to let him know about these feelings.

"It doesn't feel scary in there now."

"How does it feel in there now?"

Before I even knew what the feeling was, I said,

"Safe, Dr. Siegel. It feels safe."

It felt a little scary actually saying it. Was it safe to feel safe?

I asked him why he thought I was able to feel safe inside now.

"Why do you think?"

I knew he was going to ask me that. And—maybe for the first time in all these years—I felt like I did know the answer to my question.

"I think the states that were so sad when my mother died were terrified, and in the hospital, you helped me make them feel safe. You helped me attune to them like I attune to Sam. And I think those states, which I'd kind of lost track of—they were the last states that needed to be found, known, and integrated. Connected to. Their fear and sadness sent me to the hospital where I could be safe to do that work with you."

"And Dr. Siegel, I think the little girl states now feel seen. I think they feel safe. Soothed. I think that's why I feel safe looking inside."

We were sitting quietly taking this in. It felt good.

No more hidden fears.

No more hidden states.

"My story really makes sense. Fear is fading."

It was true. I was able to discern my present from my past.

I knew I'd been terribly afraid while I was growing up. I was not afraid now.

Dr. Siegel smiled in his comforting way. "Sounds like you're free from the constraints of your past."

It was true. I felt free.

SOON AFTER OUR SUCCESS WITH EMDR, Dr. Siegel introduced me to a mindfulness practice he was developing. He called it the Wheel of Awareness. It was an integrative practice meant to help people come to know, understand, and befriend their minds. He called it "mindsight."

As he took me through the steps, it felt like a culmination of all the work we had been doing since we first started therapy in 1991. Breathing to get grounded. Noticing my five senses and the internal state of my body. Noting how my thoughts would come and go—and the meaning I gave those thoughts. Increasing self-awareness, my ability to emotionally regulate, and my sense of being interconnected to the world.

Practicing the Wheel of Awareness was a real game changer for me. It really did give me a way to befriend the mind I'd come to feel safe in. After a few weeks of practicing it, I wanted to let him know about the remarkable changes I was noticing.

"Dr. Siegel, with the Wheel, I feel like I'm discovering a new depth of peace and freedom."

It felt amazing.

"That's wonderful to hear, Sally."

I was journaling daily. "And not just about the past, Dr. Siegel—about my present. What's going on with me now. My story."

All in one handwriting.

"I'd like to share what I've written."

"Please do!"

I read it aloud.

"*Now, I can benignly know about all the chaos, fear, terror, threats, brushes with death, wishes and plans for death, pain, all-mind-knowing, all-mind-not-knowing, all-body-knowing, all-body-not-knowing, states of adaptation. I can know the states, but I am not those states, I am only the knowledge of those states—how they came to be, how they saved me, and how they have now evolved into a story about what happened to me— about how crazy and disturbed my family was, and about how I survived it and am profoundly able to be present as I move forward in full awareness of and liberation from the prison that was my childhood...all those many years ago...finally making sense of it all."*

When I finished and looked up at Dr. Siegel, he had a big smile. It looked a little like pride. Pride in us both for all we'd accomplished.

"You know, Sally, creating a narrative of who you are is how you link your past with the present. Which is important because by linking your past to your present, you can now be the active author of a possible future."

He called it mental time travel—connecting my remembered past, my present experiences, and anticipated future.

This struck me deeply. I closed my eyes. Tears began to trickle.

"What are you thinking about, Sally?"

"My future."

"Tell me."

"Just—the future. For so long, Dr. Siegel...I've been drowning in the past...struggling to stay afloat in my present. Or lost somewhere in between. It's been so long since I've thought much about any future."

My future.

Possibilities.

Being the author of my own future.

PART 5

BY THE END OF 1998 and the beginning of 1999, there were many changes. Sam was nine going on ten, and I knew my role as his mom needed to change. He was becoming more independent—spending time with friends, involved with school, extracurricular activities, and sports. He just didn't need mothering in the same way as he had when he was younger.

Dr. Siegel was helping me understand more about childhood attachment and the way to think of my son as he was growing up.

"Do you remember, Dr. Siegel, telling Paul and me after the assessment with your team at UCLA, that Sam had developed a secure attachment to both of us?"

"I remember it well. And I believe that because of all the work you're doing—the work you have done, making sense of your childhood—Sam's sense of security will grow even stronger."

The most robust predictor of how a child will grow up to thrive, not just survive, is the degree to which that child's caregivers—the parents—have made sense of their story. True enough, I was making sense of my story, and Sam was thriving. And since his needs for mothering were shifting, I realized, *I* had to shift. I had to change my role to match his needs.

Making sense is a lifelong process...

Something else was changing—my marriage. Dr. Siegel and I were talking about it a lot in our weekly sessions.

"Tell me more about when you and Paul met."

That made me smile. This I remembered clearly...

It felt good to remember. It was 1981. I was 27, working as a talent coordinator on a talk show. Paul was a guest, introduced to me by a mutual friend. I found him intriguing...he was interested in me in a way no one else had been before. Curious about who I was at that moment—particularly about my job. He asked a million questions and asked me for some staffing suggestions for the movie he was about to shoot on location.

In those conversations, over the two days we were on set together, I thought he was the most interesting person I'd ever met. I could feel his love of life...how he was funny, energetic, and just fun. On the last day of the show, he asked me for my phone number. "I'd love to see you, Sally, when I get back from location..."

I gave it to him. I had a sense my life was going to change in a way I'd always hoped it would.

I just sat there with Dr. Siegel, remembering. It felt good to remember.

"And it did, Dr. Siegel," I told him. "Paul changed my life."

In so many ways—possibly every way—my life with Paul was the beginning of my life of actually remembering. Of having stories. Shared adventures. It was how I began to live a life full of memory and memories. It was how I started to feel connected to another person. And safe with them.

Feeling safe.

For the very first time in my life.

It began with his connections, his memories.

The stories of his life.

His very big life.

I had never known anyone like him.

At forty-seven, Paul was twenty years older than me, but that wasn't something I thought much about when we first met. I don't think he did either. He seemed ageless, and in many ways, younger in spirit than me. He often seemed to not have a care in the world, with his somewhat bohemian life at the beach, and truly lived moment to moment.

I fell deeply in love with him.

I had never had so much fun with anyone ever.

His circle of friends and family was enormous.

His family and friends were so important to him.

Paul didn't lose touch with family and friends. That had felt good to me.

My friends loved him.

He welcomed them into his world.

My world.

It became our world.

Sally and Paul.

"What did it feel like, Sally, when you first met Paul?" Dr. Siegel asked me at one point. Without any hesitation I told him, "It felt safe, Dr. Siegel. I felt safe."

And with that, I took a giant breath of relief. The feeling of safety—I'm not sure I could have described it back then, when we met. I just knew it felt like something I had never felt with another person ever, until I met Paul.

I also knew that things between us weren't quite the same now. "It's not that I don't feel safe with Paul anymore. I do. We're just not so connected lately."

Through the years of my therapy, Paul and I had drifted apart to a degree. His work was taking him away from home more and more. It's not that we were estranged—we spoke multiple times a day wherever he was. Sam and I visited him on location often. And when he was home, life was good. He was a great parent; together, our priority was always Sam. But we were changing. Both our needs were shifting. I was home with Sam in Malibu, applying to graduate school in clinical psychology. Paul was prepping his next project and was living and working mostly in Vancouver.

When Paul and I had first met, we'd been perfect for each other. He traveled for work often, and I was free to join him. Our professional worlds would also come together in the most useful way. Two years into our relationship, he was preparing a comedy film, and my experience working on sitcoms and talk shows had connected me to up-and-coming comedians and comedy writers. We became a good team.

"I was madly in love with him, Dr. Siegel."

"Had you ever been in love like that with anyone else?"

"No."

"Why do you think that was?"

We had to really work on my being able to answer that. It took a few sessions for me to sort it out.

"You know Dr. Siegel, the people I dated in LA before Paul were all very serious, and at a certain point, they wanted to know more and more about me..." I had to think for a moment—and then it came to me. "People I dated then wanted to know about my internal world."

"What was that like for you?"

"Mostly I didn't know what they were talking about."

And of course, with my unresolved history, I knew nothing about my internal world. My entire life had been built on not knowing. On keeping all internal awareness of myself at bay. Hidden. Divided states, with memory barriers. Digging deep was not something that was ever an option—and when someone wanted to get in there, or happened to get a glimpse, I bolted.

"How was it different with Paul?"

"It just was."

Paul lived so for the moment. We'd lived moment to moment. Project to project. And then we had Sam, and I got into therapy. "And then my internal world and Sam became my whole life."

I don't know that Paul had ever felt left out. He'd lovingly stepped aside for me to do the work I needed to do with Dr. Siegel and to be Sam's mom. To know myself. To be a good and healthy mom. But now...

"We've just drifted, Dr. Siegel. It's not that I've let go of him, or that he's let go of me, but we seem to be moving in opposite directions."

I sat there on the couch where I'd figured out so much. And realized something.

"You know, when Paul and I first met...one of the things that I loved about him—one of the things that made me feel so safe—was that he wasn't interested in digging into my internal world."

"What was that like for you, Sally?"

"It was great! The last thing I wanted—or even could do then—was dig deep in there."

"How about now?"

I had to pause before saying it. It was a hard awareness...but the truth.

"I would like him to be interested in what's going on with me. To know me in that way."

Another pause.

"And it's just not who he is," I said. "Like how I didn't understand when guys I dated wanted to know more about me...I don't think Paul really knows what I'm talking about now."

We sat there quiet with this big awareness of mine. Something else occurred to me.

"You know what?"

"What?"

Sam and I had just gotten back from visiting Paul on location in Vancouver.

"Visiting him there, I felt something very different between us, but I couldn't quite put my finger on it until just now."

"Tell me about it."

I just sat there. I could see what I was thinking and feeling. I was sad and I cried a little. But I wasn't confused. I knew what it was.

"In the past, when Paul was on location, wherever in the world it was, our home away from home was always that—our home away from home. This time I could feel that Paul's place was *his* home. It wasn't mine. I had no place there. Sam did, but not me."

The months to come proved it. We'd grown distant. I stopped visiting Paul on location; he was working, I was in school, and by now, at ten, Sam was old enough to make the direct flight to visit on his own or with a friend. Paul and I both knew it, felt it, but didn't really discuss it—couldn't say it.

There was still love between us. Things were rarely mean or bitter. But it was sad. Very sad. Having so many opposing feelings.

We loved each other very much...And we were both heartbroken and sad, but we knew it wasn't working.

It would take two more years for us to separate and divorce. Everything I learned in therapy helped me get through it. It was sad and painful, rarely mean-spirited. We did argue, we fought—and we knew we couldn't continue. When we finally said it out loud, when we both knew and admitted that we needed to part, something shifted. It got easier.

As I was learning more and more, the truth was our friend.

It set us free.

We were able to part friends. We've remained family all these years: Sam's parents. And, in as many ways as we grew apart, we also grew close in surprising new ways. No longer married, but lifelong friends, with a shared history. Paul, as a rule, didn't let people go—and I learned how to stay connected with him. I left, but I didn't bolt.

It became then what it remains to this day: still loving, and still a little sad at times.

I recently spoke to him about how to write about the end of our marriage. In classic Paul style, he reminded me that when we met at our lawyer's office to sign the final papers, knowing we would leave that office no longer husband and wife, he looked at me and said,

"Can I buy you lunch?"

I just love that about him.

For such a sad memory, it makes me smile even now.

I remember that as I got into the elevator with him, quiet tears trickling...I could be aware of my sadness. Regrets. Pain. Fear. *Oh goodness, am I in trouble?* I knew I wasn't in trouble or in danger—they were implicit feelings, and I knew them as such. I could know them without being hijacked by them. I was safe no matter what I was feeling.

I was happy, too...crying sad tears, but feeling happy.

Aware of it all.

As we walked out of that elevator, no longer husband and wife, and went to lunch, I knew we were okay.

Through my work in therapy, I could connect my past—being deeply in love with Paul, having a beautiful life together, and becoming the parents of Sam—to my present. Our marriage was over, but we would continue to be deeply connected in the future. Sam's mom and dad.

I was moving forward and in graduate school studying clinical psychology. Sam and I moved to a new house in Malibu close to Paul. Figuring out single life and co-parenting. I was seeing Dr. Siegel once a week.

School had always been a haven for me, especially college. Now, as a student in my mid-forties, I found it so enjoyable, and even better than it had been, without the complexities of my youth. My age was not my only advantage. I found the work Dr. Siegel and I had done to be the best preparation for studying to be a psychotherapist. Having made sense of my story and having done so under the care of a therapist who'd been so willing to see me with full acceptance, care, and safety, was certainly an asset. Not just for what I knew about my life, but, as it turned out, for what others—especially some of my teachers—didn't seem to know about their own field.

I found many instructors didn't understand DID, continuing to call it MPD. Others didn't believe it existed. Most troubling was those that did believe it existed yet viewed it as a freak show, something at best unresolvable, at worst untreatable—a lifelong prison, really. Because Dr. Siegel had couched my treatment in such positivity with the goal of healing—of making sense, resolving past traumas, allowing memory barriers to dissolve—my view of DID was that it was an adaptation to abuse, even a brilliant one, not an insurmountable deficit due to abuse. DID was what saved me. It was a response, not a trait. Dr. Siegel viewed it as a brilliant, life-saving response, and therefore so did I. I never once believed that there was something wrong with me because of it.

I knew DID was controversial. I knew there was an organization that believed it didn't exist. Still, while this wasn't easy, I never doubted the truth of my diagnosis. What I began to realize in the course of my studies was that, while Dr. Siegel had framed the therapeutic process as one of moving toward mental health and emotional well-being, for some of my teachers, the focus was on mental *un*health—on everything that was deemed dysfunctional about people with DID—almost as if healing wasn't a goal, much less a possibility. It seemed that some simply didn't believe it was a real condition. Nor was it a condition with any viable therapeutic treatment.

It made a huge impression on me, making me ever more thankful to Dr. Siegel for showing me that DID was completely treatable—that resolving the many traumas of my childhood would lead to the dissolving of the memory barriers that were at the heart of DID, and allow me to be completely free of the complexities of DID while maintaining all the knowledge of what my childhood was and the valuable wisdom it affords me to this day, especially as a therapist myself. His treatment led me to integration—to the linkage of differentiated parts. The pursuit of mental health and emotional well-being had always been the guiding force of my work with him—and of my training as a therapist, and of my work with clients now. It was about always looking for what was possible. It was about breakthroughs, not just breakdowns.

THERE WAS ANOTHER AREA that bothered me. In a class on early childhood development, the instructor said: "We're so lucky now to have an entire research group of children who suffered great early deprivation—Romanian orphans. And in them, we're seeing the effects of such early deprivation. These children will never be okay."

Lucky? Never?

Again, it seemed psychotherapy was all about mental unhealth. This instructor had no way of knowing what the long-term effects of the early deprivation of Romanian orphans would be, as it had not even been ten years since they had been discovered post-revolution. And why were we so confident in predicting what children would never or always be?

True, Sam was developmentally delayed by a few months when we first brought him to Dr. Siegel—but he caught up in less than a year, which was well documented by the UCLA team tracking him. By this point, at age ten or eleven, he was more than okay. He was thriving.

I raised my hand to offer a new perspective, hoping to share Sam's story, but no sooner had I than the instructor shut me down: "That simply isn't possible," she said. Developmental theory told her what was possible and what wasn't, and there was no arguing with it.

I didn't argue. I just sat there in disbelief, realizing many of my instructors—therapists themselves—seemed so rigid in their beliefs and teaching. Sam's progress was living proof that developmental theory is not set in stone. And I remembered how, in therapy, Dr. Siegel would often come in with new research, ideas, and new ways of thinking—always open to possibilities. I promised myself then that as I progressed in my education, training, and practice, I would remain open with curiosity to new ideas and the current research.

I was becoming more interested not just in early childhood development, but also, specifically, in adoption. There didn't seem to be an abundance of evidence-based research about the experience. What did it mean to be adopted—to experience what Sam had? He was struggling with it now in a way he never had. We'd always told Sam he was adopted, and we'd talked about it a lot. But it seemed now to be affecting him in a way I didn't yet understand. Kids at school had been telling him that adoption meant his dad and I weren't his real parents, and I could see that that really bothered him.

I tried to reassure him: "Oh no—I'm your real mom. Daddy's your real dad. The lady in Romania was the person who gave birth to you."

We went through a few weeks of Sam acting out in a very particular way. He began taking money from his dad and me without asking. One day Sam and I were at a surf shop looking around, and he asked if he could get a skateboard. When I said, "Not today, Sam," he said, "But I have the money."

And he pulled three twenty-dollar bills out of his pocket.

"Where'd you get that, Sam?"

His face had gone blank as he showed me the sixty dollars; he didn't have an answer. I wasn't sure what to think, what to do, or how to talk to him about it further. While I didn't understand the cause of his behavior, I knew a lot had been written about this kind of acting out with adopted kids Sam's age. So, I knew it wasn't a case of bad behavior. And I'd learned enough from Dr. Siegel not to get hijacked by the thought *Sam has to learn right from wrong.* I knew it would be better for me to make sense of it, so I could help Sam make sense of it.

Just a few days after this, I attended a workshop on adoption where adult adoptees spoke. It was so moving and enlightening, offering me a whole new perspective. The speakers shared how, as children, it was confusing and hurtful when their adoptive moms avoided or discouraged any mention of their biological mothers as "real" moms. It helped me realize that for an adopted child, it's natural to wonder about where their life started before adoption. And it wasn't a child's job to hold back their curiosity about where they came from. How their story began. Nor was it right for me, as a parent, to be defensive in the face of this curiosity, as understandable as it had been that my instinct had been to assure Sam vigorously that I was his mom. It was our job, as the parents of adopted children, to attune to their inner world, and to help them attune to it too, helping them make sense of their story. And it was always up to the parent to understand their child's struggles, never the child's job to understand ours.

I literally rushed home that afternoon. When I arrived, Sam was in a real state. Our babysitter—who didn't know what had been going on—had seen Sam taking money from my drawer and given him a consequence. Sam had gotten so angry he broke a bracelet of mine and tried to flush it down the toilet. When Paul came over and heard what happened, he got angry at Sam. By the time I got there, poor Sam was curled up on my bed, just staring at the wall.

That same blank look on his face.

I sent everyone home and went to sit with Sam.

"You know Sam, it's never okay to take money from anyone—you have to ask."

"I know, Mom."

"But I have to tell you something."

I told him what the adult adoptees at the workshop had talked about. He sat up, looked straight at me, and I saw tears rolling down his face. It clearly meant something important to him.

"I'm so sorry, Sam. I was completely wrong to tell you that I'm your real mom. I'm your adoptive mom, and your Romanian mom who gave birth to you is your real mom. I understand your wanting to know all about her. I want you to know all you can."

So odd that no one objects to calling a child adopted, but often there is an unwillingness to calling the parent an adoptive mom or dad. I realized in that moment the reason Sam called me his adoptive mom was because...I *was* his adoptive mom.

The truth will set you free.

I got up, went to my office and got the file with all of Sam's adoption documents. I showed it to him. Again, we'd told him from the start he was adopted. We'd even talked about going to the orphanage in Romania. But we'd never told him the name of his birth parents. Now, I showed him his Romanian birth certificate, with their names on it. And the name they had given him. Francisc. He recognized it because we'd named him Sam but kept Francisc as his middle name. I sat there with him for some time. He was crying. Silent tears. Right before he fell asleep, I told him,

"You know, Sam, we don't know how to reach your birth parents. We don't have their address. But if you ever want to write them a letter, I'll help you keep it safe so if we ever find out how to contact them, you can send it."

With that, Sam fell asleep.

The next morning at the crack of dawn, Sam woke me up to read me the letter he had written his birth parents:

Dear mom and dad,

My name is Samuel Francisc Maslansky. You don't know me. I'm your son. I'm in the fourth grade. I live in Malibu, California. My dad is Paul, he's a movie producer. My mom is Sally, she's becoming a psychotherapist. My parents are divorced now. I never got to meet you. I want to meet you as soon as I can.

The letter went on to talk about his pets, his friends, his school... his life...his story. He signed it, "Love from Sam, your son."

It was the most beautiful, heartfelt thing I'd ever read. I realized immediately that he was making sense of his story. His recent acting out was because I'd confused his story. I was his adoptive mother. And now, he finally knew the name of his birth mother, too. This was when I realized how I'd mistaken *Sam's* adoption story for my own. I had told him the story of what it had been like for me to adopt him. Now, he was hearing and reading about his own story from the documents. Writing his story in the letter to his birth parents. Sharing his experience. His feelings. Making sense of his story. And letting me hear it. I heard it. It was an incredibly transformative moment for us both.

No more taking money without asking.

No more breaking things.

The feeling of making sense.

Double breakthrough.

In 2006, I would see that look on Sam's face one more time. He was seventeen—the summer before his senior year in high school. We traveled to Romania as volunteers at an orphanage. We were both nervous and excited. Approaching the front door of the orphanage the first day, I could see Sam as he saw the many little faces pressed up against the window. As he walked up the stairs ahead of me, he stopped. A little wobbly. Face ashen, that blank look. For a moment I thought he might faint. But he gathered himself together and went, very slowly, through the entrance.

Over the next few days, Sam said little to me. He was very engaged with the other young volunteers and with the children, particularly one little girl and boy. He spent lots of time with them. It was a side of Sam I'd never seen. Deeply compassionate and caring, in a way only children really bring out in you. He was mesmerized by them. Understood them. The entire experience seemed to give him answers. After a while he told me that as he entered the building that first day the smell hit him hard—he recognized it:

"And Mom, as I walked in, I got this flash of me in one of those cribs looking out, and I was overwhelmed with a feeling I finally figured out was despair."

He told me it was a feeling he'd felt before and never understood. He was glad to now know where it came from.

Implicit.

Making sense...and of his story, not mine.

IN 1999, WHEN SAM WAS IN FIFTH GRADE, his teacher noticed he was struggling. An educational assessment revealed some learning differences. As he moved into sixth grade, it became clear the school wasn't equipped to support his learning. Paul and I began a search for a school that could. Coincidentally, the best choice seemed to be a school located near Chapel Hill. It had a very positive, cutting-edge approach. Paul, Sam, and I talked at length about what to do, and after consulting with Dr. Siegel, Sam and I moved to Chapel Hill in 2001 for him to attend that school for seventh grade. I took a leave of absence from my studies, Paul visited regularly, and we spent holidays and summers in LA. I continued to meet with Dr. Siegel as needed by phone.

In 2003, at the end of eighth grade, all agreed Sam had received the help he needed, and we headed home to LA. I completed my master's degree and began an internship as a marriage and family therapist (LMFT) at a training clinic in Beverly Hills. The opportunity to share my education and the insights I'd gained with Dr. Siegel with clients for the first time confirmed this was exactly what I was meant to do. I loved working with clients.

BY NOW, DR. SIEGEL had published two bestselling books: *The Developing Mind*, a foundational textbook for interpersonal neurobiology (IPNB), the transdisciplinary framework he developed, integrating many fields including neuroscience, psychology, and attachment theory; as well as *Parenting from the Inside Out*, coauthored with the child-development specialist Mary Hartzell, which was informed by IPNB. He had also begun offering small group classes in IPNB at his Mindsight Institute in Brentwood. I was interested in joining one of those groups. As we discussed the possibility of bringing my therapy with him to a close—since I no longer needed weekly sessions—I wasn't sure what he'd think about me becoming one of his students.

So, I asked him. He was fine with it, as long as I'd be comfortable seeing him in a new role. And I was—ready to transition from being his patient to his student. Eager to continue learning all I could from him.

We also talked about me attending a workshop on memory he was offering soon. He suggested I find a seat close enough to the front so we could touch base.

The day of the workshop, I found an aisle seat, and when he arrived, we were able to connect. What happened next was one of the most profound therapeutic experiences of my life.

He was talking about how memory is encoded—implicitly and explicitly, getting into the details of the brain, mind, and memory. An attendee in the back asked him a question. I can't remember exactly what she said, but she wanted his opinion on how false memories were encoded.

The false-memory movement had gotten a lot of attention over the previous ten years. I hadn't given it a lot of thought, as I believed it to be misguided and simply wrong—as did Dr. Siegel, who was outspoken on the subject. Just as I don't remember exactly what she asked, I don't remember his exact answer. What I do remember is precisely how his answer made me feel. In the most compassionate manner, he made it clear that he didn't agree with the false-memory theory and, through his review of the research, effectively conveyed his point.

When he finished speaking to her, he shifted his gaze, looked straight at me, and nodded.

I was overcome with a feeling so strong and exhilarating that it caught me by surprise. I'd never felt anything like it before. Before I knew what'd hit me, I remembered Dr. Siegel describing to me the feeling of being attuned to as the feeling of feeling felt. I felt *felt*.

It was amazing.

IN 2005, SAM WAS A SOPHOMORE IN HIGH SCHOOL; I'd finished grad school and was working toward licensure. I was studying with Dr. Siegel and absorbing everything I could about IPNB, attachment, neuroscience, trauma, and mindfulness. Much like my experience in grad school, many supervisors at the clinic I'd been training at didn't recognize two things that had been essential to my healing and recovery: mindfulness and EMDR. These practices seemed to be dismissed by many out of simple ignorance about them, even though by then there was a substantial body of research backing both. Being aware of this lack of even curiosity by so many with authority in the field made me more determined to learn all I could about mindfulness and EMDR and what they could do for those who'd experienced trauma. In addition, the way my supervisors and other authorities I came to know at the clinic spoke of DID reflected none of my experience. I was not yet brave enough to disclose my experience as a counterpoint, but I could feel my dissatisfaction mounting.

It was especially frustrating that I was barred from teaching clients about the Wheel of Awareness and any mindfulness. The argument, again, was that these methods were too obscure; the supervisors at the clinic wanted me to rely on the tools everyone else was using. But the Wheel and the mindfulness practices I'd been taught by Dr. Siegel had been complete game changers for me, as much as any of the work we'd done to dissolve memory barriers. The longer I practiced with these tools, the more grounded and connected I felt. And the easier life got—even when it was hard. I'd discovered the concept of equanimity too, which meant mental calmness, composure, and evenness of temper, especially in difficult situations. Equanimity became my goal. To this day, I practice the Wheel daily.

IN JANUARY 2008, I MOVED BACK TO CHAPEL HILL. When Sam and I had moved for his schooling in 2001, I'd fallen in love with the place where I'd spent part of my childhood. And slowly, across the five years I'd been back in LA, I'd realized I didn't want to live there anymore. Having long now made sense of and resolved the trauma of my childhood, the past no longer haunted me. In my time in Chapel Hill, I'd reconnected with friends I'd grown up with, and hiked through the woods on trails I'd blazed with my dog as a kid. I marveled at some good memories the town held for me. What's more, Sam had graduated high school in 2007. He was now in college on the East Coast. That too gave me the freedom to return to North Carolina.

Once back, I began building a private practice. As a licensed LMFT, I enjoyed working with individual adults, families, couples, and parents, and the variety of issues they brought to therapy. I had a special affinity for working with adoptive parents. Helping my clients make sense of their own stories was always where I began. Of course, within these populations, traumas of all sorts showed up, and I went on to train in many modalities and techniques designed to respond to it: EMDR, attachment-based EMDR (EMDR focused specifically on relational trauma experienced in early childhood), the Adult Attachment Interview, or AAI (a research instrument that assesses individuals' recollections and how they have made sense of their own childhood experiences, which can be used clinically to gauge how clients' early attachment patterns influence their behaviors in the present), and mindfulness-based stress reduction, or MBSR (which uses mindfulness to teach people how to manage stress and improve their well-being). My studies with Dr. Siegel and IPNB continue to this day, culminating in my joining him in his course, "Understanding and Treating Disorganized Attachment and Dissociation," in 2022 and 2023, where we discussed the therapy we did together. I've never worked directly with a DID client, but I often work with clients whose partners have DID. When I first started out, I wasn't sure working with DID clients was within my scope of practice, but found my expertise in supporting their families.

After moving back to Chapel Hill in 2008, I also connected with my best friend from elementary school, who'd been visiting from out of town. We were fifteen last time we met; now, we were in our fifties. I was curious about what she remembered about my family. Without giving her details, she told me she didn't remember being at my house much—we mostly hung out at hers—but she'd been afraid of my dad, and she knew how afraid of him I was. I told her about my memories, my therapy, and DID. A few months later, she called to tell me there was something she'd never forgotten—or truly understood—until I'd told her a bit about the work I'd done in therapy so many years later. She said she'd been at my house, in maybe fifth grade—when we were ten or eleven. It was raining, we were bored, and I asked her if she wanted to play a game called rape. She said she didn't know how to play that. I told her, *you just lie down on the bed, and I'll lie on top of you and bounce up and down.*

WHEN SAM FINISHED COLLEGE, he first went back to LA, eventually moving to Galveston for a job. There he met the woman who would become his wife, Maria, and her daughter, Gigi, soon to be his step-daughter. Living life.

One morning my phone rang.

"Hi Sally."

I recognized the voice immediately. It was my fifteen-years-older brother. I hadn't heard his voice in nearly twenty years.

He would be in the area the next day, could we have lunch?

I said yes and invited him over.

"See you tomorrow."

I wasn't afraid. I wasn't nervous. I didn't shut down. No fight, flight, freeze. I was curious and open.

"We don't need to talk about anything that happened..." were his first words to me. We sat at my kitchen table, caught up a little. Just a little. He got right to his point. He was worried he hadn't been a good parent to his two adopted children. He'd read some blog posts I'd written for *The Huffington Post* on adoption parenting, and he wanted to pick my brain.

We spent a few hours together, which I was happy to do. At one time, I'd felt close to him. I'd liked him. Now I felt compassion for him, because I could see he was a tortured soul. We said we'd stay in touch, and we did, mostly by email.

About six months later, on a Sunday morning, I got a call from his sister-in-law letting me know he'd just committed suicide. He'd shot himself in the head. It wasn't exactly shocking news. Nothing about that family—my family—could really shock me any longer. I didn't feel so much a loss, either; the acute loss had happened long ago. But it did have me reflecting on the legacy of having grown up in such a disturbed family. And it reminded me that I was certainly not the only one who'd suffered. I felt a sadness I hadn't felt before. I was sad for us all.

About three weeks after his death, I received an email from his daughter. She introduced herself by asking, did I even know she existed?...and did I know her dad had killed himself? Then she went on to tell me that, a few weeks before his death, she'd gotten a letter from him saying one day soon, she might find the need to reach out to someone for support. He told her to contact his sister Sally—even though she didn't know me and had always been told I was crazy. "You don't need to talk to her about why we've been out of touch. But she knows a lot about adoption, and she'll be able to help you."

She said she didn't understand what it meant. Could I bring any clarity to it?

I wrote to say that her father had come to see me, and he'd been curious to hear what I knew about adoption. That he'd worried he hadn't been a good parent to her or her sibling. I let her know how sorry I was for her loss, how clear it was how much he loved her, and if I could help, to please reach out.

She never did.

More things came to light over the next few years about how disturbed my family was. It didn't make me happy to know these things, which were extremely sad. However, they were validating in a way I hadn't known before. I guess you could say that what I learned brought me some closure.

A YEAR AFTER SAM AND MARIA WERE MARRIED, they decided to relocate to Chapel Hill. I'd never expected it, but was delighted by their news. When the three of them arrived, Gigi, Maria's daughter, was just starting the seventh grade. Their intention was to stay with me and get settled with their jobs, and Gigi's school, before finding a place of their own. Then the COVID-19 pandemic struck. In one way, it was a good thing for us all—cohabitating suited us.

One morning Maria came to tell me she was worried...Sam was having trouble standing up. I went with her to check. He couldn't stand up because it made him dizzy. Maria needed to get to work, so I cancelled my morning clients and took Sam to the ER.

As we walked in, he could barely hold his head up. They took him right in to see the doctor. He texted me in the waiting room, almost immediately, to say they were giving him an MRI.

The next thing I knew, Sam was texting me a picture—there was a giant tumor at the base of his brain.

Oh my god. There's something wrong with Sam.

Breathe, Sally, breathe. No mind wandering. No hijacking allowed. Bring your attention back to what is happening right here, right now. Breathe. Get grounded. Discern past from present. Something's going on; we don't know exactly what yet. Equanimity. Breathe. Call his doctor.

I got his doctor on the phone immediately. She was seeing the same picture I was. The first words out of her mouth:

"It's not cancer."

Thank God.

Breathe.

"What is it?"

She explained that it was an acoustic neuroma—vestibular schwannoma—a non-cancerous tumor that grows along the cranial nerve, which was responsible for hearing and balance.

Bringing into my awareness: *benign. Not cancer.*

Breathing. One-breath-at-a-time. Breathing in...and breathing out, with a huge whewwwwww...

Sam's doctor went on to say that the ENT surgeon she wanted Sam to see was waiting for him at his office. Just then, Sam came into the waiting room. He was remarkably grounded, telling me exactly what his doctor had told me. Not cancer. Going to meet the ENT surgeon right now.

Grounded.

He was very present, not in any way shut down. And I worked to keep my worry to myself, to attune to Sam.

I had a huge impulse to ask him if he was all right.

I knew he hated when I asked him that.

I kept my worry to myself.

Breathe. Slowly.

We drove to the ENT surgeon's office, which was nearby. COVID protocols meant I couldn't go in with him. So, I was waiting in the car, working on staying calm. I didn't make any calls. I was very aware that Sam was an adult, and he was married to a wonderful and oh-so-capable wife. This wasn't about me. I was here to support Sam and Maria.

I'm not sure how long he was in with the doctor. As he got back into the car, I asked, "How can I help, Sam? What can I do?"

"I don't know yet, Mom. I want to talk to Maria about everything... I'll call Dad to let him know."

He was clearly upset with the news, but remarkably strong and grounded. I recognized he was being flexible in his thinking. Curious, open, accepting. He was taking it one moment at a time.

"I've an appointment to meet the other surgeon in two days...I'll find out more then. I think they want to operate right after Thanksgiving."

Don't forget to breathe.

Sam did meet with the other doctor two days later—a neurosurgeon who would operate alongside the ENT surgeon. He came out of her office seeming okay. They had scheduled surgery for the first of December. About ten days away. During their meeting, she let Sam know that she and the ENT surgeon and their team were very experienced. They'd done this exact surgery many times with great success.

"It's a really big tumor, Mom," Sam said. "The doctor told me my surgery would take eight to ten hours. All in all, I'll be in the hospital about a week."

Breathe.

OVER THOSE NEXT TEN DAYS, we all got ready. Paul was flying in. Two of Sam's closest friends from out of town were planning to come too. My friends rallied around. Maria's family and friends as well. We were surrounded by love and were holding each other close.

A few nights after the ER visit, I was sitting on my bed, reflecting on everything. I hadn't cried once since the diagnosis, and suddenly my entire body began to shake from the inside out and tears flowed. I didn't panic. I welcomed it. I knew my body was doing what it needed to. I didn't give it any negative meaning. It wasn't a warning of danger. It wasn't a memory. It was simply my nervous system responding to what was happening here and now, and to all I'd been holding inside the last few days. I let it unfold. It didn't last very long. I slept well that night.

We went on to have a small, quiet Thanksgiving—just the four of us. Extremely thankful. The next day, Sam and a friend went to a hockey game. Two nights before surgery, Paul arrived, and Sam picked him up from the airport. The night before surgery, we had a quiet dinner. And then, it was the day. Maria and I woke up early with Sam to take him to the hospital. Because of COVID, only two people could be in the waiting room. Paul opted to wait at the house.

We arrived at the hospital by 5:00 a.m. At around 6:00 a.m. a nurse came out to say we could—one at a time—go see Sam. Maria went first, then me. Sam was sitting in a pre-op area, sporting a hospital gown, shaved head, and a COVID mask. I could see the stress in and around his eyes above the mask. I knew he was scared. I stood there with him for a few moments. I knew that if I allowed myself, I could really let loose and cry my eyes out. But Sam would hate that. So, I kept my tears to myself and hugged him.

"I love you, Sam."

"Love you, Mom."

I love you so much, Sam.

In the end, Maria and I would be in the waiting room for eighteen hours—not ten. The nurses gave us updates every few hours. At around 2:00 a.m., both surgeons finally came out to let us know they'd finished. They'd been able to remove the tumor, but they'd had to sever Sam's acoustic nerve, so hearing in his left ear was gone. Maria would spend the night in the ICU with him. I was heading home. As I walked out of the waiting area, Sam was being wheeled to the ICU. I could see that he was still intubated, but he opened his eyes and saw Maria. He reached his hand out for her.

As anticipated, Sam spent a week in the hospital. When he came home, he faced many challenges. I don't believe any of us—Sam included—realized that because of the severed acoustic nerve and the balance issues, he would have to learn to walk again. He was in a wheelchair for quite a few weeks, and he was in physical therapy immediately, working hard on walking and recovery.

I was amazed by his resilience and perseverance. He never gave up.

Nearly two years later now, Sam still faces challenges with balance and his hearing loss. There are days that he does get frustrated. Overall, though, he's doing well. Working. Seeing friends. Spending time with his wife and daughter. Going to the gym. And luckily, through it all—he never got COVID.

I have rarely ever known anyone so emotionally well-balanced. His strength and courage take my breath away.

"You know, Mom," he told me once, "I know I may struggle with some things the rest of my life but I'm happy to be alive, and I can handle it."

A remarkable human being.

ONCE THINGS SETTLED DOWN, I reached out to Dr. Siegel to let him know what had happened. As always, he was amazing and helped me process it all.

"Do you remember, Sally, what brought you to therapy with me in the first place?"

Of course I remembered.

"My fear that there was something wrong with Sam."

"What do you think of that now?"

It took me a moment to gather my thoughts. They were not confusing or confused. They were not hiding. They were right there for me to see, feel, and know.

"I think that when Sam first discovered the tumor, I immediately knew he was in trouble. But I wasn't disorganized in my thinking. I didn't get hijacked by fear or anger. I could know it, see it, feel it, and remain grounded in the knowledge that whatever it was, he would get through it."

I would get through it.

My feelings about it all made complete sense.

"I think I've developed that 'bring it on' attitude," I told Dr. Siegel.

With a big smile, Dr. Siegel said, "Yes, Sally, I think you're able to be aware of anything now without moving out of your window of tolerance into chaos or rigidity."

He took a little pause here and then added, "I think your parenting of Sam has given him that stance as well."

I believe that's true, too.

Before we closed our Zoom session, I told him about a time, a few years earlier, when Sam and I had been together on his birthday, and something had happened that made me emotional. I started crying a little bit while Sam remained just as steady as ever. I'd asked him then why he thought he was so much more balanced with his emotions than I was.

"You know what he said to me, Dr. Siegel?"

"Tell me."

"He said, 'You know what, Mom? I think it's because I had a better mother than you did.'"

That brought some tears. Happy tears.

Finally, everything made sense.

THE END

ACKNOWLEDGMENTS

FIRST OF ALL, I wish to thank the participants in Dr. Dan Siegel's Mindsight Institute course, "Understanding and Treating Disorganized Attachment and Dissociation." Your thought-full questions about my experience of DID and how Dr. Siegel's treatment was so healing truly inspired the writing of this book.

To those who so graciously provided their expertise and support early on—Joy Elliot, Mary Kalbach, Dr. Mary-Anne Kate, Vivek Khare, Paul Maslansky, Sylvie Rabineau, Beth Rashbaum, Fred Schepisi, Maria Shriver, and Lynn York—your insights were so valuable. I thank you all. And thanks to the members—therapists and clients—of the Attuned Psychotherapy Trauma Recovery Group for inviting me to join you. It has been an honor, and I appreciate all we have shared together.

At WME, my thanks to Gail Ross, for your valued advice and guidance to this new world of publishing for me, and for finding just the right home for my manuscript. And to Cameron Dames—thank you for your instant belief, enthusiasm, and assistance.

At New Harbinger Publications, to Elizabeth Hollis Hansen: your belief in *A Brilliant Adaptation* and thoughtful and kind guidance set everything in motion—I'm so grateful. And to Vicraj Gill, for your careful and insightful editing—your attention to detail and care for my words made this a stronger book. To Amy Shoup, for your inspired art direction and just the perfect cover.

To Maria and Giselle—I am deeply grateful for all that you bring to Sam's life and through him, to mine. I so appreciate your insights about my book and thank you for sharing your impressions.

To my cherished and steadfast friends from the many times and places in my life—Ella Beirith, Jenna Best, Kasey Blaustein-Greener, Clare Brown, Suzanne Browning, Donna Collins, Margee Eife, Elizabeth Emerson, Elizabeth Gabler, Lisa Kay Gist, Michael Grimsley, Stella Hall, Ann Clark Howell, Lesli Johnson, Robin Johnson, Sandy Lieberson, Beth McCauley, Mary McCoy, Michelle McCumber, Jane Ridlon, Norma Safransky, Mary Schepisi, Sue Smalley, Stephanie Smith, Rene Sparrow, Melanie Woods, Dey Young, and Stephen Young—you have all supported me when I have needed it most and offered much needed and appreciated feedback as this story unfolded for me. I thank you so very much for your friendship.

To my lifelong dearest friends—Mary Chancellor, Judy Gordon-Cox, Cindra Ladd, Sarah Lieberson, and Mary Jane Ufland—thank you for being with me through both the darkness and the light as I lived this story. Your support never wavered. Your love and your belief in and excitement for *A Brilliant Adaptation* has meant more than I can say. You lived so much of it alongside me, and that made all the difference.

For Paul Maslansky—though you are now gone, I will cherish forever the journey and adventure of it all—especially as our beloved Sam's mom and dad. Your enthusiasm and encouragement every step of the way for *A Brilliant Adaptation* means so much. Thank you for everything.

To my son, Sam—being your mother is my life's deepest privilege. Having your loving support and input in the writing of my story—which naturally overlaps with parts of your story—has meant the world to me. Thank you for all you do and are.

Dr. Dan Siegel, your knowledge, wisdom, compassion, and guidance transformed my very being. As my lifeline for those many years, your unwavering belief in my healing shaped not just the resolution of my childhood trauma, but how I live and work today. I'm so grateful and wildly fortunate to have had you first as my therapist, then teacher, and now colleague and friend. In every way, without you, this book would not have been possible. Thank you for being you.

And to my clients, who over these many years have been a constant source of learning, inspiration, courage, and transformation. I thank you all for the work we have done together. I love being your therapist.

Lastly, to Maverick, my sweet, gentle, soulful companion of fourteen years. You were literally at my side for every word I wrote. Your quiet, grounding presence steadied me through it all. Losing you now, just as I complete this process, breaks my heart. I dedicate this last line of the book to you, my dear boy. I will *always* remember you.

SALLY MASLANSKY, LMFT, has been in private practice for twenty years in Chapel Hill, NC. She treats families, adoption, trauma, parenting, and adult individuals. Her training is in interpersonal neurobiology (IPNB), mindfulness-based stress reduction (MBSR), eye movement desensitization and reprocessing (EMDR), dialectical behavior therapy (DBT), adult attachment interview (AAI), attachment theory, polyvagal theory practices, mindfulness, and the wheel of awareness practice.

Foreword writer DANIEL J. SIEGEL, MD, is a noted neuropsychiatrist, executive director of the Mindsight Institute, and associate clinical professor of psychiatry at the University of California, Los Angeles David Geffen School of Medicine. He is author of The Developing Mind, The Mindful Brain, and other books, and is founding editor of the Norton Series on Interpersonal Neurobiology.

MORE BOOKS from
NEW HARBINGER PUBLICATIONS

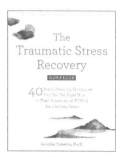
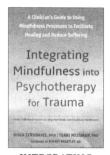
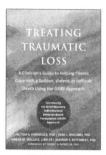
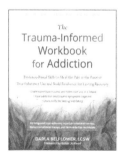
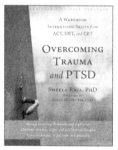
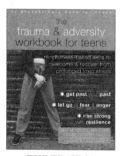